"I love the message that Ken [...] way he uses his life journey to share how powerful your mind is and how it can work for you to break free from traditional beliefs is amazing. I look forward to witnessing many Ungraduation ceremonies as people not only read but apply the call to action."

—Robert Raymond Riopel
International Best-Selling Author of *Success Left a Clue*,
App Designer, and Life Transformational Trainer

"The human desire is to avoid pain and to seek pleasure. Most choose their path in life unconsciously, and in many cases are not "happy" with the results they are currently experiencing. In Ungraduated, Ken Hannaman leads you to the explorative journey of your inner being . . . the part of you that you may not have ever contemplated before. He uncovers universal principles, belief systems, and the mindset to find purpose and meaning in life. The most important question in life, in my opinion, is "Who Am I?" and in Ungraduated, you will be able to put together the puzzle pieces of the answer to that question for yourself."

—Gunther Mueller, Founder of DreamLifeMasters.com

"As a fellow misfit who needed an education in the school of hard knocks, I am so grateful that Ken Hannaman gives us in *Ungraduated* the gift of seeing a bold new way to approach everyday life. This guide toward self-discovery is chock full of actionable, bold, and thoughtful insights that can only come from a well-studied and well-lived life."

—Vincent Pugliese,
Author of *Freelance to Freedom* and *The Wealth of Connection*

"As someone who is obsessed with connection, I can say that there's probably nothing more important than connection with yourself! Ken does an amazing job giving people a plan to make tangible changes in their lives to cranking!"

—Chris Tuff
Author of *USA Today* Best-Selling Book
The Millennial Whisperer

Free Gifts for You

UNGRADUATED
LIVING & LEARNING
A PODCAST WITH KEN HANNAMAN

UNLOCK YOUR Mind

Go to www.ungraduated.com now
to sign up to receive your gifts.

Ungraduated Living & Learning podcast
is available on your favorite listening apps
and at www.ungraduated.com/podcast

Ungraduated

Finding your why & dropping out of outdated belief systems

Ken Hannaman

Ungraduated: Finding your why and dropping out of outdated belief systems

© 2021 Ken Hannaman All rights reserved.

ISBN 978-1-950721-18-4

Published by Harshman House Publishing

Scriptures marked NIV are taken from the NEW INTERNATIONAL VERSION (NIV):
Scripture taken from THE HOLY BIBLE, NEW INTERNATIONAL VERSION ®. Copyright© 1973, 1978, 1984, 2011 by Biblica, Inc.™. Used by permission of Zondervan

Contact

Harshman House Publishing
P. O. Box 82
Spring Valley IL, 61362

Dedication

To my best friend, soulmate, life partner, amazing woman, and wife Crystal. . .

My Ungraduation in life began with you.

Little did I know in May of 1998, upon laying eyes on you from behind the counter of my then entry level, minimum wage job at Taco Bell in New Kensington, PA, that you would have such a profound impact in my life.

Our lives have at times have felt like the first line of the Charles Dicken's novel, *A Tale of Two Cities*: "It was the best of times, it was the worst of times." We have had far more moments that we've lived in our best of times, but through the darker days, you have been by my side undeterred.

To think, had that stop light not stayed red just a few seconds longer at the corner of Freeport Rd and Route 356; everything in our lives would be different. So much happened at that crossroads of our lives. I met you there and almost lost you there.

You never gave up on me, though so many times I gave you every reason to. You have helped form me into the man, leader, and human being that I am today.

I will forever be indebted to the universe for bringing you into my life. The two of us together is proof positive of serendipity and synchronicity.

Each time I gave you a reason to run, somehow, you stayed. Thank you. I needed you far more than you needed me.

As you know, my love, everything in life happens for a reason. It's just taken me a little longer to figure all those reasons out…

Thank you for being the woman, wife, best friend, and life partner that you are for me. As exciting as our lives have been the last 24 years, not a day goes by that I don't awake with the same zest and exuberance for life—because you are a part of it.

I love you with all my heart, and thank God every day that I get to experience this thing we call life— with you in it.

With enduring love for all of eternity…

"Kenny"

Contents

Foreword 1

Preface 5

Part 1
Seeing & Believing 15

Chapter 1
Blind Spots 17

Chapter 2
Seeing Through Our Labels 29

Chapter 3
Seeing the Laws, Obeying the Laws 41

Part 2
Personal Abundance & Growth 59

Chapter 4
The Thirst for Knowledge 61

Chapter 5
Getting Your Mind Right 71

Chapter 6
Generating Personal Abundance & Happiness 79

Part 3
The Connection of Body & Mind 91

Chapter 7
Self-Synchronization 93

Chapter 8
Thinking Yourself Healthy 105

Chapter 9
Manifest Your Life 113

Part 4
Taking Action & Living Your Purpose 125

Chapter 10
The Power of Belief 127

Chapter 11
Finding Purpose & Mission 139

Chapter 12
Living an Ungraduated Mindset Daily 149

Epilogue & Ungraduation 161

Acknowledgments 163

About the Author 167

Endnotes 169

Foreword

My journey with Ken Hannaman began via a LinkedIn message on October 26, 2017:

> Hello, Tommy.
>
> I heard of you through a mutual friend, Sam B. She works with our marketing team. We had a pretty good conversation recently while she was in the Cleveland area visiting my market. Wanted to connect. I think we may have a great deal in common.
>
> My best,
>
> Ken Hannaman

That message now seems like a lifetime ago. Ken's message to me is also a great opportunity to remind us to never hesitate to reach out to someone we want to meet, know, or build a relationship with. The worst they can say is no or simply not respond. We never know where a warm introduction will take us in this oh-so-precious and short life of ours. But sometimes, it takes us exactly where we're supposed to go—from friendship to fellowship to pure goodness. This is how I felt about my dear brother Ken Hannaman, whose Legendary book, *Ungraduated*, is now in your hands.

To say our journey together over the past few years has been an epic one would be an understatement. Like Ken, I am a seeker, consummate learner, and relentless pursuer of all things truth. Through countless book recommendations and hundreds of texts containing universal wisdom, a true friendship of respect, love, and authenticity has been born—all traits Ken exudes each and every day of his life.

Ken has asked me to speak to his Corporate Executive Team, is a Founding Father and senior member of my Legendary Life Mastermind, and has spoken to my entire Legendary Life Community on the insights of his book, *Ungraduated*.

He doesn't just talk the talk; he actually walks the walk and practices all of the wisdom and tools from his book on a daily basis. He now has graciously bestowed these simple tactics on us in order to Ungraduate from our old, damaging, and completely useless ways of thinking that hold us back from achieving the life of our dreams.

You now hold in your hands a world-class playbook on how to master your thoughts, rewire your heart from scarcity to abundance, and live a purpose-driven life of joy and generosity.

Are you ready to transform? Are you willing to accept a new challenge and adventure? Are you ready to lean in and do the simple tasks to build and live the life you were born to have? If so, this is the book for you. I absolutely love this line from the book, which is a teaser of the results you'll achieve if you follow Ken's guidance:

> "You will see that the old societal belief system banded down to you is what is keeping you shackled in mediocrity."

Damn! Like most of this book, that nugget of wisdom hit me right between the eyes and was exactly what I needed to hear when I read it.

Warning: *Ungraduated* is not for everyone. If you are certain of your views and opinions, are closed-minded and unwilling to hear new perspectives and ways of thinking, then go ahead and put this book down. This book is for open-minded seekers who are constant learners.

The more we travel, learn, and read, the more we realize how little we know. I consider myself very open-minded and agreeable to new ways of thinking, and Ken challenged even me during certain parts of this book. Wait until you get to the out-of-body experience chapter and hear Ken's and other's stories of out-of-body travel while they were sleeping. Wow. It will truly blow you away. I'm not sure I'm quite ready for sleep travel yet—LOL.

My hope for each of you is that you take the wisdom of this book with an open heart and mind and apply it to your life. My secondary hope is for you to enjoy and underline as much of *Ungraduated* as I did. If you do, you will truly Ungraduate from antiquated ways of thinking and step into the person you were born to be and the life you were meant to have. Here's to all of us living the life of our dreams and being the amazing people we were born to be.

As always, Carpe Diem and Be Legendary, my fellow Beautiful Humans!

Tommy Breedlove, *Wall Steet Journal & USA Today* Best-Selling Author of the book, *Legendary*
Founder of the Legendary Life Mastermind & Movement

Preface

"The unexamined life is not worth living."
~Socrates~

There is so much more to life than meets the eye. We often only see what we are told to see. Not nearly enough of us go deeper into the depths of self-discovery to form our own belief systems. Our lives are lived within the framework of a system that has been set up by a society that wants us all to fit neatly into its objectives. We often look at external forces we think are the big drivers of our lives versus inward at our own abilities and ways of thinking that deliver our outcomes.

Often, we meander through life using an old mental operating system. We don't realize the program we have been given limits our potential. Unfortunately, we haven't been taught how life really works. Much of the studies and discoveries in today's science are beginning to show how our own mental energy and thoughts generate the outcomes of our complete existence—our health, wealth, happiness, purpose, and overall experience in life. The time has come to upgrade to a new operating system so that we can live life to its fullest potential.

The teaching and lessons within this book are designed to work backward to help you rethink your passions, purpose, and overall happiness in life. As you read on, the goal is to see what old belief systems and teachings you may be holding on to that often hold you back from achieving more. My mission and purpose in including my personal experiences is to help you *Ungraduate* from limiting life systems that you may not be aware you are operating with. By the end of this book, my sincere hope is that you will see and experience life differently.

You will begin to see that the old societal belief system handed down to you is what is keeping you shackled in mediocrity. Through the Ungraduation process from these old belief systems, you will find the empowering ability to fulfill your life's potential and purpose in more ways than you have ever dreamed. As you read on, you will see life in a way that hasn't been brought to your attention before. It will be your own personal Ungraduation to new beginnings and opportunities to live life to its fullest.

My Story

I prefer to take the humble approach to life and divert attention away from myself. While I crave purpose and meaning, I am quite bashful in the spotlight. Those who are closest to me may not know this about me, but I am an introvert at heart. I am always examining my own thoughts, life, beliefs, and reason for being. For as long as I can remember, I have been an individual who attempts to seek out the answers to life's biggest questions:

- Why are we here?
- What is our purpose?
- What happens before birth and after death?
- What is consciousness?
- Do we have a soul, and what exactly is it?

While I don't have the answers to all these questions, I have made a great deal of progress in my own learning and have started to find answers. The experiences and truths that I have discovered compel me to share the information that has benefited me in my life's success. The truths that I unearthed have changed my life for the better and propelled me to achieve both the personal and professional goals I have sought to attain. By stepping back and peering through the looking glass at my life, I discovered the connectedness of our thoughts and beliefs to the impact they have on the results in our lives. I found the power that we each possess to change our lives for the better and to put ourselves in the driver's seat to all the achievements and successes we desire in life.

What I have found to be the case in my life, as with many others, is that we do not realize the veil over our eyes that keeps us from seeing the truth: that we direct our outcomes through our belief systems. The power of our thoughts generates our beliefs, which then in turn produce most of the outcomes in our lives. This belief system takes many different forms. It often begins with our parents, then our education systems, and eventually society helps round out our life views.

The big misconception many of us are encouraged to believe is that *life is random*. We begin to think that *life happens to us, versus because of us*. The material in this book is designed to show us how that belief is a myth. This book will walk readers through the eye-opening perspectives and scientifically backed evidence of the connectedness we have to our thoughts and how those thoughts either entrap us in life or set us free. Our thoughts have this effect on us as do much of society's indoctrinations that we've picked up along the way.

Much of life that we live today has become a mental prison that cements us even more into a less-than-empowering posture. Throughout this book, I will go in depth about how this occurs due to the many distractions and deterrents of our everyday lives. The great news is that upon recognizing these traps, we can learn to avoid them and grow our personal awareness and life empowerment. As we become more Ungraduated from the old learnings, programs, and limiting belief systems, we will begin to realize our highest and truest potentials in life.

My Childhood Journey

My life story begins like many others. I was born into a low-income household to young parents who barely had enough money to take care of themselves, let alone an addition to the family. Since my parents were of Christian faith, they believed they should "do the right thing" and get married since they had a child. Thirteen months after I was born, a little brother joined our little family in our new journey together. My parents thought they weren't prepared for one child, and they now had two.

My mother and father did the best they could to care and provide for us, but I remember it being hard. They tried to make their relationship work, but the love for each other just wasn't there. They tolerated each other as much as they could and would often work to recommit after a bad fight, but the days of holy matrimony were numbered. At around the age of five years old and not completely understanding, I watched as they decided to divorce.

Like many separations, it wasn't pretty. While I didn't completely understand at the time, I never held it against either of my parents. My mother forged on and did her best to provide for us after a difficult divorce. I know it was hard on my father as well. So much so that he landed in a mental institution soon after the separation. My brother and I didn't see my father while he received the mental help and rehabilitation he needed to return to a normal life.

Eventually, my father would gain visitation rights to spend time with my brother and me. It felt like years before this new arrangement took place. When I finally did see my father again, he was a shell of his former self. The visits were often short and awkward. To this day, I give him credit as he wanted to see us, but my brother and I just didn't see him as the same person we once knew. The visitations would follow an on-again, off-again pattern for a few years. At one point, I remember them stopping altogether.

My mother remarried when I was around twelve years old. In my stepfather, she had found a man who would provide her with the love and attention she felt she deserved, and she hoped he would provide the father figure she believed my brother and I needed. My father eventually remarried as well after the successful completion of his rehabilitation. By the time my brother and I were adolescents, we found ourselves splintered between families, each with a new stepparent.

Although it took getting used to, I loved my new stepfather and stepmother. As a young adult, I was able to tell that my mother and father each seemed happy in their new relationships. Besides, who was I to decide for them whom they should spend the rest of their lives with? I was not concerned at that point in my life with what they each wanted. I know my parents did the best they could, but I was determined to escape the poverty, stress, lack, want, and need that I had become so accustomed to in my early childhood.

The Highs & Lows of Adolescence

At the age of seventeen, I got my first job: a minimum wage, fast-food position. I loved that job so much that it began to take precedence over my schooling. At that point in my life, I found myself in a very awkward position. While I had enjoyed most of my time in school to that point, I found myself beginning to dread school. In fact, I started to despise it. I can't recognize the precise point in time when this began, but it was somewhere around my sophomore year in high school. Most of my childhood, I had received good grades and was on the honor roll and at times high honor roll. The days of earning any type of honors recognition regarding education and learning quickly began to fade.

Throughout elementary and middle school, I had been rather popular and accepted at school. This began to change in high school. Quickly, I found myself more and more excluded. The more popular kids weren't including me in their groups. I had been relegated to the average group or even worse, the outcasts. To this day, I don't know what caused this to happen, but I found myself unwilling to face school due to the new and awkward category I found myself in.

I began to skip school. Missing a day here and there turned into missing a week here and there. It got so bad at one point that I had missed twenty-one days of school in row. At the time, my mother was working days and nights trying to make ends meet. Even if email and electronic report cards had existed to notify parents how their children were doing with attendance and grades, I don't know if she would have had the time to stop and check.

To top it all off, I had discovered freedom thanks to my job, as I was able to (barely) afford a new car and insurance payments to legally drive it. This newfound passport to freely roam city to city came with new possibilities. Quickly, I was able to escape my current situation for what I deemed to be far better surroundings. The problem was that at the time, my mental state was not the best. The problems I was having in school were causing me to have more of a rebellious spirit. I found more in common with outcasts and people who I believed were more like me. I began finding companionship and acceptance in people who were involved in more sinister daily activities.

I didn't feel that I was actively seeking out trouble, but trouble often did have an ironic way of finding me during those later adolescent years. The people I was associating with were doing and selling drugs. I found myself interested in fitting in, so why not take up similar actions? There would be long nights of binge drinking, smoking marijuana, and other not-so-great extracurricular actives. I don't remember how we acquired this stuff, but get it, smoke it, and drink it we did.

Often, our evenings would progress from a neighborhood house or apartment and into the streets. If you think what we were doing inside was bad, it certainly didn't get better when we went out roaming the streets. One evening, a few of the kids I was with decided they were going to break into cars and begin stealing car phones. Yes, I said car phones because this was the late 1990s when cell phones were still essentially car phones. I don't have a good answer for why we did this—probably because there just wasn't anything else to do. I remember how awful doing that felt, but there was an element of a rush to it. I would find myself routinely participating in this activity when hanging around some of the same kids. Even though there was a psychological rush to it, I just seemed to go along with it just because the rest of the kids did it.

The exhilaration of stealing something eventually turned into the despair of being caught. One evening, some alert neighbors saw us and called the police. That singular event could have changed my life forever if it had just happened a few weeks later. I was weeks away from being eighteen at the time, so the police considered charging me as an adult. Ultimately, I evaded that catastrophe and happily accepted my juvenile court case with a guilty plea and a sentence of community service and a parole officer who would follow up with me.

While this part of my life remained mostly camouflaged to the outside world, I continued to find meaning and purpose at work. My fast-food friends accepted me with open arms. Most of the high school kids who were working there didn't know me, as they didn't attend my school. I found it much more enticing to be a part of my work clique rather than going to school to face the degrading challenge of fighting to be recognized as cool. Plus, I was being paid to go to work, and I wasn't seeing any revenue coming in from attending a high school that I detested more and more as the weeks and months went on.

My life was quickly spiraling out of control before it even really had the chance to begin. By the time my junior year of high school was over, I had missed more school than I had attended. I remember seeing my report card the end of that junior year. The failing and incomplete grades had replaced all of the A's and B's I had earned as a child. I was mortified, embarrassed, and disappointed in myself. I told myself that I would make the effort to recommit and get back on track my senior year.

That opportunity was abruptly cut short. About three months into my senior year, I was called into the guidance counselor's office. My parole officer was there too, and this seemed to be something that had been scheduled without my knowledge. It was explained to me that due to all the school I had missed the previous year, I would have to repeat the eleventh grade. I asked about summer school—if I could finish all my classes my senior year and make up lost credits in summer school, could I still graduate with my class?

The answer was an abrupt no.

"Don't you see all the incompletes and failures you have from eleventh grade," the guidance counselor asked pointedly. "You can't just make those all up in one summer semester."

I knew that was the case but didn't want to accept the fact.

It was mid-December of 1999, and I had recently turned eighteen years old. It was in that moment in the guidance counselor's office that I made another life-changing decision. I glanced back and forth between my parole officer and the guidance counselor and said, "I'm dropping out."

My parole officer snarled back, "You can't—by law you have to finish."

By law? What law?

He began going on and on about something pertaining to the crime I had committed, and I had to finish high school in order to make good. I recognized he was bluffing. There was no law I was aware of that said I had to finish school, even with the actions I was found guilty of as a juvenile. I remember pulling out my driver's license in a pretentious manner to show them proof of my age and that as of December 4, 1999, society legally had to recognize me as an adult. I was free to make my own decisions at that point in time—for better or for worse.

I again looked at them both and said, "I'm leaving, and you can't stop me."

As I got up and turned to leave the room, my parole officer mumbled, "Good luck making it in life flipping burgers." It was one last attempt to shame me and make me feel like more of a failure. It worked.

Inwardly humiliated by what I was about to do, I walked out of that guidance counselor's office, down the hallway toward the exit of the school to the parking lot, got in my car, and never looked back.

The Here and Now

Those early days of adolescence seemed to have melted into oblivion as I've since lived through my twenties and thirties. As I embark upon what I believe will be another great decade of growth and learning having recently turned forty years old, I can't help but look back and be filled with gratitude for how my life turned out.

As I write this book, I am still in the restaurant business— twenty-three years later. I am responsible for leading 300+ company restaurants and overseeing 400+ franchise restaurants. I get to lead and interact with hundreds of thousands of individuals throughout the course of my professional responsibilities.

On top of my corporate executive responsibilities, I am venturing into my own passions around entrepreneurship as I seek to share my life learnings and successes with others in the hopes that they too can reap the rewards. All of this I take great pleasure in.

I am blessed with the opportunity to lead and influence a multitude of people and share learnings with them with every interaction. It is the single greatest joy I receive from my current position. I certainly don't take my role in leadership lightly, and I realize the opportunity I have been granted to leave long-lasting positive impressions on the people I meet every day. I also realize that what I do is not really that important.

In the grand scheme of life, I am simply a passerby, just another person who is hoping to make a difference in the lives of others. I don't take myself too seriously as I have come to understand that what I do is not about me. I have learned that to receive, we must first give.

It is in service toward others that I have decided to write this book. I have lived through places of self-doubt and incompetence. Fear and uncertainty at one point ruled the day. Feelings of inadequacy sparked a mental state of resentment, need, and constant want for more—more of what I did not know, only that I felt that getting more would bring me into a better mental place. I was a person who craved and needed status to feel as if that would bring me fulfillment. Through some of the self-development, learnings, and mental reconditioning I have developed, I wish to share these perspectives with others who seek the same purpose, meaning, and self-driven success in their lives.

While I am just an average individual, I have watched my life transform into *anything but average.* My journey has taken me from a high school dropout earning minimum wage and teetering on the brink of complete failure, to a position of fulfillment, meaning, purpose, success, and happiness. The best part of this all is that I am experiencing these examples of success in all the major aspects of my life:

- Personal relationship with my wife
- Personal relationship with my family and loved ones
- Financial success, freedom, and happiness
- Physical and emotional well-being
- Purposeful meaning beyond myself and my family
- Spiritual significance
- Creation of good luck and good fortune

I could probably continue with that list, but I think you get the point. I have discovered that by changing my mental programming and belief system, I am now in control of my life. What happens in my life happens *for me* not *to me*. I have effectively learned how to shift my mindset from that which was a *fixed mindset* into that which is a true *growth mindset*.

The most profound learning in my life has been that we are conditioned to believe we are not in control, that we are not powerful in our own regard—to believe we are inadequate. Much of this comes from those who are close to us, but it comes from society, too.

To break free of these limiting beliefs, we must begin the internal work. It is not an easy process, but it is possible if you have an open mind. I can assure you that this process works. But it does take an open mind and a level of commitment to the practice of mental reconditioning.

For me, this reconditioning occurred over time and required a lot of introspection. It has taken me more than ten years of my life, but it doesn't need to take you that long. There are simple daily practices that you can implement, then watch results begin to follow. I liken this reconditioning to an *Ungraduation* of sorts—a way to step back and regain control of our own minds and challenge the beliefs that others have hardwired into our systems.

You'll find in this book the necessary thought process changes you'll work through to untangle the old limiting beliefs put in place through family upbringing, schooling, religion, government, media, and even our careers. You will discover what is necessary to change your thought patterns about many different topics in life and to ultimately generate a new graduation of empowerment and abilities to drive your life toward ultimate fulfilment, happiness, and success.

I hope you are excited to form new belief systems and move onward into new, empowering ways to live with purpose along the path to true happiness, fulfillment, and success in life. Keep an open mind and analyze everything from a fresh perspective to the best of your ability. It's OK to question what you first read. You don't have to take it all at face value. Do your own introspection, and just simply allow this information to sit with you and resonate.

It's time to begin the *Ungraduated* process of removing old limiting beliefs and starting to see the world through eyes in which we generate our life's outcomes, individually and collectively. We are at the wheel. We are in control, and we can manifest our best and highest potential. If you are willing to take a step back and study your life, thoughts, and beliefs closely, you will find that it certainly is a life worth examining because it is a life worth living!

Part 1
Seeing & Believing

Chapter 1
Blind Spots

Two fish are hanging out together as they notice a third fish approaching them.
The third fish says to the other two as he passes by, "Hey! How's the water?"
The two fish give each other a perplexed look.
"That's a strange cat right there," one says to the other.
With that response, his friend follows with, "Yeah. What's water?"
~Source Unknown~

As humans, we don't live in water, but we rarely walk around asking each other, "How's the air?" Are we any different from the gilled and finned ones who live in water? The air is obviously just as important to us for survival as water is to fish. We live within an environment where we do not necessarily see the air, but we know it's there.

Much like humans with air and oxygen, do fish ever ponder the fact they live within the vastness of water? They do not necessarily see it, and they quite possibly could be so oblivious as to not even think it to be there. But make no mistake: they live within it, and it is vital to their survival. Whether they can see it or comprehend it, the water in which they reside is the very source they depend on for much of their survival.

The air is obviously just as important to humans for survival as water is to fish. We live within an environment where we do not necessarily see the air, but we are aware of it. What we often do not stop to realize is that there are also many levels of energy that cycle through and overlay the physical environment in which we reside.

We usually don't see this energy or perceive it as being there, but these different forms of energy most certainly do exist around us. Just as with the air, we cannot see most layers of energy with our eyes, but they most certainly exist.

What other connections are we missing through not having the deeper awareness to see our environments for what they are? What else are we missing about life? Could there be far more that we are connected with than meets the physical eye?

Allow me a quick moment of digression back to one of my favorite childhood series, *Transformers*. The popularity of *Transformers* is likely greater now than it was when I was a child thanks to the blockbuster movies that have been created in recent years. However, long before I was watching Shia LaBeof befriend Bumblebee on the big screen, I was watching Optimus Prime battle it out with his archnemesis Megatron. The principal concept of the cartoon-series-turned-Hollywood-blockbuster is *there is more than meets the eye.*

Much like in *Transformers*, we are going to uncover the realities that do exist beyond our vision and that lie hidden beneath the surface of what we as humans perceive as the real world. For much of humankind, the real world has remained tucked away and hidden beyond the awareness of our physical senses. Many of us are like fish, unaware of the water. It is a major human blind spot. We are unconscious of what our source of life truly is. Once we uncover our realities for what they are, the illusions of life become apparent. Many of these illusions are self-perpetuated. Unknowingly, we limit ourselves and our potential in life because we "can't see the water."

Once we understand the connection of our physical life to the elements of energy that exist beyond our physical senses, we begin to open a new world of understanding. When we deprogram ourselves of limiting life beliefs, a new empowering way of living begins. It is through this deconstruction—or as I prefer to call it, "Ungraduation" from old beliefs, indoctrinations, and social programming—that we truly begin to live life to our fullest human potential. Happiness, meaning, purpose, fulfillment, financial success, professional success, and anything else that you deem important in life begin to flow your way in abundance.

Seeing the Water

We live in and are a part of an amazing field of energy that binds together the entirety of the Universe. Scientists have proven that the physical matter that composes everything from the planets and galaxies we can physically see, down to the tiniest particles of energy only amounts to about 4% of the physical space that occupies the known Universe. So, what composes the other 96%? There have been many speculations throughout time.

There is a well-known but failed experiment that attempted to prove that empty space between all physical matter was filled with what was described as ether. The thinking was that just as waves move through water and sound moves through air, there had to be some medium in which light moved through empty space. The belief was known as the luminiferous, (i.e. light-bearing) ether. The experiment was known as the Michelson–Morley experiment, and was conducted in 1887. [1]

The experiment involved studying how the Earth moved around the sun. With that movement through the empty space between the two, what should be produced was thought to be what was termed "ether wind." Because the researchers could not verify the presence of this ether wind, the test concluded that there was no known ether or ether wind that exists in the empty space of our Universe. Until recently, this became the generally accepted principle within the scientific community.

In 2012, science made one of the most significant discoveries of the modern era. Scientists rejoiced at the news that it had been proven there are particles of energy that interact within empty space with other electrons. These particles that interact within the quantum space within the void of physical matter are known as the Higgs Boson particles. The name of the field of energy, that was previously thought to be empty has been dubbed "Higgs-Ether" or the Higgs Field.[2]

The Higgs Field exists within every space of the Universe, meaning that which appears to be empty and even overlying space is territory occupied by energy. The omnipresence of the Higgs Field is what affects all known elementary particles that contain mass within the entire Universe. This proves energy is everywhere. It's all around and within us.

The fact is "the field," as I'll refer to it, has always been here. Science must operate within a means to which all must be based on fact. Facts are what science is based on and precisely why science is important for the major discoveries of our time. Careful and meticulous effort based on fact is put in place in order to prove and disprove theories. What the proving of the Higgs Field has given science is the answer to a long-misunderstood measure of reality: we are not separate from the Universe, and evidence now proves it.

Humankind is part of the Universe, but we are also connected to every part of it—to all things that represent other forms of physical matter. We are connected to everything from the stardust of the galaxies and solar systems down to the minerals that make up the matter of the Earth . We are intricately interwoven with each other and all things from the fabric of the Universe. We may not see it, but we can feel it if we begin paying attention. This is how we begin seeing our blind spots.

Have We Been Duped on Evolution?

Is it possible that we have been programmed to incorrectly believe survival comes down to those that are the fittest? Could it be that we are actually wired to coexist and lift our weakest up with those that are stronger? We've been taught that life is a game of "survival of the fittest" and that we live in a "dog-eat-dog world." But what if those beliefs were really off base and just a matter of our own misunderstanding?

From around the time that the Michelson–Morley experiment was dubbed a failure, Darwin's theory of evolution was being released. Darwin produced his conclusion that the world and all its species are in constant conflict with each other. His theory essentially states that the world and its creatures are all in a constant battle of survival of the fittest in which only the strongest survive. This theory created a lens through which much of today's worldview is still seen—that we live in a winner-take-all type of environment. We have literally been groomed and programmed to believe that this is how nature operates. However, in more recent times and with new and modern technology, humankind is beginning to challenge Darwin's theory. Evidence is surfacing regarding our ability to alter not only our bodies' chemical makeup and genetics, but also the potential to alter and change our own biological conditions.

> If we focus our completion on Ourselves, real progress is made. For meaningful progress, run the race against you.

We are learning that our bodies and minds don't need to take tens of thousands of years to alter for the better. We have the capability to make changes to our biochemistry and nervous systems with just a few minutes of focused thought per day. Suddenly, it no longer remains that survival depends on the strongest and fittest among us, but rather those who are self-aware can survive and thrive![3]

No Such Thing as "Mindless Thought"

There are many medical examples of patients who had been diagnosed with terminal illnesses and given just months to live, only to completely alter and change their life outcomes. Within a few months, these medical miracles are given clean bills of health. Cancer tumors vanish at times with enough individual focus and mental mind shifts from the loving and caring thoughts of individuals within the circles of these patients. How can the stories of these miracles simply be coincidences?

Might it be possible that we are literally thinking ourselves into our own unique life circumstances? There are brave scientists presently who are beginning to break out of the shackles of old thinking and belief systems and now are portraying that we as humans are a bridge to the physical and nonphysical Universes. We exist in both a mental state and a material state with each overlying the other. Talk about a major blind spot that most of us truly have yet to see!

We are beginning to realize that we are not victims of circumstance. Instead, we are the creators of much of our existences, which in turn become the realities of our everyday lives. "As above, so below" is a saying that rings true in this example. Each thought we put out into the Universe becomes the beginning of possibility. The stronger we dwell on these things, the more they begin to materialize.

Have you ever stopped to think about the power of your own thoughts? We all would be well served to do just that.

Our thoughts, both positive as well as negative, project out into the Universal Field of energy what impacts us on an individual and a collected level of human consciousness.

The programming we receive over the years largely states we operate on an individual level, only impacting each other when we encounter one another. The implications of this belief system have led us to believe we are not interconnected as a human species. We have been raised to believe that we function within a standard set of rules in nature and that we are in competition and separate from one another. The evidence is mounting in undeniable ways that we impact ourselves and each other with our thoughts and the energy that we put out into the field through every moment of time.

Tuning in to the Broadcast

The reality we are discovering is that we as individuals are indeed a part of the whole. This fact has been a major blind spot for humanity. We live within a reality of cause and effect. What one does will not only affect him- or herself, but also the larger collective source of energy. Take for example the countless stories of parents feeling and knowing that their children are in danger. Thousands of miles may separate them, yet they can *feel* that something has happened. Intuition, as it has been called, works on these energy channels of communication.

So often, this sixth sense has been tossed aside as "coincidence." How many coincidences must we ignore before we realize the substantiality of the evidence being presented?

Radio waves are constantly being broadcast all around us whether we see them or not. It is not until we turn on the radio and tune to a specific station that we hear them. Should we continue to be naïve enough to refuse to see that the communication of the quantum Universe works in the same fashion? All we need to do is attune ourselves with the right mental state in order to receive the answers that we so desperately desire in life.

Here is the amazing part of this reality that is being uncovered: whether we attune ourselves to the broadcast or not, we are still putting out into the Universe our thoughts, beliefs, and desires through every waking moment of our lives. Our brains are acting like receivers. The Universe is the conduit through which those signals are received. Humanity is like 8 billion individual cell phone towers broadcasting thoughts across the globe and out into the Universe.

> Intuition is available to everyone. There is no special person or religion needed; we simply have to become attuned to receive it.

Those broadcasts bounce off each other, out into the Universe, and then right back to the receivers in our heads—our brains. The scary part about this for most is that we have been asleep at the wheel for a long time. Most of us have not known that we are generating our own realities one thought at a time. The empowering part of this discovery is that we can take back control and become master architects of our lives, bringing into existence some of the most magnificent realities we could imagine.

All we need to do is become the observer of our thoughts. That is the first step to bringing our thought energy back together with our physical bodies. Our thoughts and our physical realities are forever intertwined. There is no way to separate them. The ticket to the magnificent dance of life and all we could ever desire is to become aware of the signals we are broadcasting. What are the hourly, daily, monthly, yearly messages we keep beaming out that eventually come back to us?

Each of us is generating a broadcast every moment of our life. Is your broadcast more of a negative and pessimistic radio show, or one that is enlightening and full of possibility? If you were on the receiving end of that broadcast, would you tune in even more because you felt a positive connection that could empower you, or would you want to change the channel quickly due to the bad vibes you were picking up?

These are the signals that make up who we are every day of our lives. These signals don't define our lives on any given day, but over the course of weeks, months, and years, we become the type of signal we've been putting out. We become it because after we think it, that signal brings back to us the same type of energy. Like attracts like—this saying was created for good reason. It is not simply a figure of speech.

Seeing Yourself into Reality

As I step back and observe my life, I can honestly say I have figured out part of the secret to getting what I want. Years ago, I used to be an individual who *wished* for the things I didn't have. I would aspire to gain the things I wanted such as a nicer car, house, more money, better health, etc., but I rarely *saw* myself with those things. I wanted them all, but they seemed too far into the future. There is a big difference between dreaming of your future success and seeing yourself *with* that success *now*.

What we have to remember is the profound reality that we only ever truly live in the present moment. That is why our thoughts in the present moment matter so much. How we think of ourselves every moment of the day leads us toward our future. We can never really escape the present moment. So that is why our thoughts in each present moment matter so much, even if we are thinking of the past or future. No thought we exude ever happens outside of the present moment.

I know what you're thinking: how can I see myself with these future things if I don't have them now? That is one of the belief systems we must address and change. In order to attain what we want in the future, we must see ourselves living that reality now. It does require a mind shift, but it is possible to make happen. Allow me to walk you through a real-life situation I recently experienced.

For so much of my adult life, I allowed myself to place the "I'm too fat" label on myself. My bathroom mirror reaffirmed this every day of my life from my early twenties into my thirties. I lived with this daily broadcast signal of "too fat" for nearly twenty years. I put that signal out into the Universe multiple times a day, not just once when I was looking in the mirror after a shower, but many times throughout each day. It was a major blind spot for me. As if my thoughts weren't bad enough, the reflection I saw helped me cement it into my mind. Over the years, my body reaffirmed the position my mind had taken for it. I began to gain weight.

The irony of how the field works is this: it gives you exactly what you put out into it. Every thought you broadcast comes back to you. If you think you are fat, you will begin to receive reaffirming ways that will most certainly keep you fat. You'll find more reasons to live a lifestyle that is not conducive to weight loss. Even if you have some short-lived attempts at diets and exercise, you will likely find yourself back at square one.

It's why so many diet plans don't work. In the present moment, we see ourselves as fat even as we diet. We have to change the signal we are putting out before we will get the results we want.

I began to balloon up from about 160 pounds at the end of high school up over 190 pounds as a young adult. By the time my thirties had come around, I was well over the 200 mark, and I topped out at around 250 pounds in my late thirties. I can assure you, it was not a weight gain as a result of building muscle. I had packed on some serious fat, and it showed. This didn't occur from sitting around lazily each day doing nothing but watching TV. I was active. I would exercise at times. I would diet and eat right at times. I even tried many different forms of diet pills. I would achieve some short-term wins with some weight loss here and there, but in my mind's eye, the image I saw reflecting back at me was that of being too fat. Nothing I did to seemed to work.

Seeing, Therefore Being

At Christmastime in 2019, I decided to approach things differently. I had done research on the mind–body connection and decided to take a new approach. It began with me telling myself that I loved my body. That's right—my body and I had a reunification of love and appreciation for one another. I decided right then and there that the year 2020 was going to be different for me. I was done looking with disgust at the image I saw in the mirror. The morning of December 26, 2019, was a turning point. That day, I saw a young, vibrant, healthy body that had supported my soul and aspirations for the previous thirty-nine years of my life. I looked myself in the eyes and said out loud, "I love you. Thank you for allowing me to enjoy these last thirty-nine years." I also made my body a promise that day. From that day forward, I would do my best to take care of and provide it with the proper daily nutrition it was designed to take in and give it the physical activity required for continued optimal performance. I looked myself in the eyes that day and said, "I am healthy, and I am in shape. My body is strong and vibrant."

Those words became a daily mantra for me. No more blind spots for me in regard to my health and well-being. Not a day has passed from that point and through the writing of this book that I haven't upheld my end of the bargain. I've been perfect on daily exercise, and with cutting out soda, deep-fried food, and almost all meat from my diet (I'm still eating fish at the present time). While the sugar part hasn't been perfect, it is most weeks. I'll provide a sugary sweet here or there for my body as a reward to my ego for doing well overall. But for the most part, my thoughts have been aligned with "I am healthy, and I am in shape. My body is strong and vibrant."

Thinking those words each day keeps me from any temptation that might pull me off course. I cannot and will not allow my physical actions to sway me from the personal commitment I made for myself. Even though some days would go by in 2020 that I saw myself in the mirror and was tempted to think differently, I wouldn't permit myself. I continued to persist in the present moment of that very challenging year broadcasting that I was fit, healthy, and in shape. Even through all the shutdowns and reasons that would give most people to not work out, I excelled, and my weight loss did as well.

I averaged a weight loss of two pounds each week, ten pounds a month, and sixty pounds in six months. The mental image I put in my mind was seeing myself on my scale with the numbers 190 looking back at me. That is exactly where I sit months later. I have maintained that weight and am currently framing the mental image in my mind that "I am strong and have a good muscular tone. I will maintain a healthy 190 pounds while building more muscle." This daily thought has led me into doing push-ups every day. I started at twenty push-ups the first day and have built in one more rep each day.

What began as barely being able to do twenty push-ups now has resulted in my doing more than one hundred each day. My arms and chest muscles are becoming more defined. My body is becoming what I have wanted for more than twenty years, and it has been achieved through a daily focus and *seeing myself as I am*. Not wishing myself into the future but telling myself each day, "*I am* healthy." I achieved more change in six short months than I had accomplished in twenty years, just by shifting my thoughts.

The two most powerful words in the English language are *I am*. They are powerful for that very reason. They reaffirm your existence. Think of all the moments you say, "I am." You say it in the present moment, and it reaffirms the words that come after— one . . . day . . . at . . . a . . . time.

Objects in Mirror Closer than They Appear

Lincoln Steffens (April 6, 1866–August 9, 1936), was a journalist who lived through industrial rise and economic prosperity in America. He was not just any journalist; he was a Muckraker. Theodore Roosevelt developed a negative connotation of Muckrakers. In a speech given on April 14, 1906, he compared the Muckrakers to a passage from John Bunyan's *The Pilgrim's Progress*, "The man with the muckrake . . . who could look no way but down."[4]

In basic terms, what the twenty-sixth president of the United States was trying to say was that Steffens only focused on the negative and never the positive. While this may be true from Roosevelt's seat at the table, it was required from Steffen's position.

Steffens saw blind spots that many others weren't seeing at the time. He wrote about the many levels of political and economic corruption as well as the social pitfalls that were a result of the many big businesses and corporations that were rapidly growing in America at the time.

Steffens was also ahead of his time in regard to parenting and education. Well before America was engrossing itself with equal views on men and women, he was advocating that, "The father's place is in the home." This was not a popular view at the time, as men were largely seen as the breadwinners and providers for their families and often left the women to care for children and the home. At the age of fifty-eight, he got to practice what he preached with a welcomed but unexpected birth of his first child.

At the age of sixty, Steffens wrote a letter to his then-two-year-old son, Pete, that focused on finding oneself in the unknown. He was an outspoken opponent of formal education and an advocate for the need to keep a child's curiosity levels open rather than allowing them to be programmed and told what they should or should not believe. In this letter, he writes:

> An educated mind is nothing but the God-given mind of a child after his parents' and his grandparents' generation have got through molding it. We can't help teaching you; you will ask that of us; but we are prone to teach you what we know, and I am going, now and again, to warn you: Remember we really don't know anything. Keep your baby eyes (which are the eyes of genius) on what we don't know. That is your playground, bare and graveled, safe and unbreakable.[5]

When we look back in the rearview mirror of our own life, what objects, realities, and beliefs stand out to us the strongest that we have grasped onto so tightly? Let's look at these beliefs and see them for what they are. Who gave them to us? Did we take them as truths without doing our own research? What if these so-called truths are only at best theories of others on life?

Let's see the blind spots for what they are and work together to Ungraduate from the limiting life beliefs that have shackled us to mediocrity or worse. Remember what it was like to look at the world with childlike wonder? Pull your attention away from that rearview mirror no matter how large the objects may appear. There is a great reason why the rearview mirror is small in comparison to the windshield: we have a lot more to see in front of us than we do behind us. Onward we go!

Ungraduated Call to Action:

- What are some of your blind spots in life? What areas of self-discovery to you want to learn more on and understand?
- Are there any beliefs you have in life that you are questioning right now? What are they, and what specifically are you seeking to understand more about?
- What is one thing in your life that you were misled regarding and later discovered that you had been misinformed about or were never given any information in the first place?

Chapter 2

Seeing Through Our Labels

"Throughout life, we are put into boxes to categorize how people see and know us. This is how stereotypes originate, because people would rather read the labels on the box instead of taking a look and seeing what's inside."
~Gaby Rodriguez~

Who am I? My name is Ken Hannaman. I am a husband, business executive, leader, and writer who was born in a town northeast of Pittsburgh, Pennsylvania. By my count, that is four labels: my name, marital status, career titles, as well as where my life began on planet Earth . In any introductory conversation, these labels are being generated, assumed, and pondered over. This is simply an example of what happens when we interact with people who are new to us. But are we these labels?

It may certainly be true that these are the labels society has neatly rounded out for us to describe what it is that defines the human experience in physical form, but let me assure you *we are not these labels*. We may need these titles to function in our current society, but our true nature goes far beyond simple words that aim to define our lives. Because we live in a society that operates under titles and labels that we use to define ourselves as individuals, we have been programmed to believe that these categories are who we are. The layers go even deeper when we begin to understand that we are generating a sort of self-talk in our mind of who we are. But more on that later when we dig into the power of belief in a future chapter.

The Real Me

Will the real "me" please stand up? While there has not been any evidence found through science or religion of a soul, I believe that is what we are at the absolute center of our existence. I believe we are pure energy consciousness, part of the whole or Source (God, Universe, higher selves, the divine, the sacred, etc.) who created us. While we may never see the soul in X-rays or find it on any type of body-scanning instrument, I do believe the soul or a part of it is harnessed and anchored within us. This soul or conscious energy is what is guiding the physical instrument we use to interact in what we know as physical life. The body is the vehicle or a bridge between that of the nonphysical realms of existence and what we experience here on Earth and within our daily physical existences. We exist both physically and non-physically. We are never separate from God or the Source, of which we are a part.

What a beautiful gift to have been given when you really sit back and think about it. We are eternal energy at our core, but we have been given the opportunity to experience what a physical life is like. We are forever intertwined as part of this continuum. I am not Ken Hannaman: husband, business executive, leader, writer, etc. I am the consciousness inhabiting this physical form who is leading it through these temporary physical experiences.

When we look at so many of the historical spiritual teachings, the messages are there for us, but they are often hard to comprehend or understand. Our ancestors spoke and communicated differently, often in allegorical ways to avoid persecution and ridicule. They tried to leave clues for us as they too were figuring out what they were and their purposes for existence.

My aim here is not to dissect the many religious teachings. Rather, I want to try to explore the perspective that while we are most certainly not God, it is my belief, through my own truth experiences, that we absolutely indeed are connected with that Source and can direct our lives here on Earth through that connection.

It takes a conscious understanding, realization, and effort to put the practices into place that can empower us, through connection with our Source, and direct our lives where our consciousness (higher selve) intends us to be. Decluttering and removing the barriers, labels, beliefs, and old programs placed upon us is part of that awareness and a driving force behind accomplishing this goal.

If not Labels . . .

If not labels, what defines us? Becoming self-aware helps us to realize that we are not the collective sum of the items we have accumulated over our lifetimes. We are not our clothes, cars, houses, money, hobbies, and other aspects of what society has taught us to believe we are and what define us. I am not advocating that we disregard our accomplishments and interests in life, rather just that we do not allow them to be part of what defines us. There is nothing wrong with having goals and aspirations in the physical world; that is part of the experience. It is when we constantly aim for these physical aspects of life as our main points of gratification that we will quickly find ourselves lost and longing for the next fix.

We have all experienced this at one point or another in life. How many times have we wanted that latest and greatest piece of technology? How about that new car that you remember having bought and promised yourself you would keep in pristine condition because of how proud you were to have attained it? A short year later, it becomes just another item in your life as you are longing for the next physical accomplishment that you believe will bring satisfaction.

I believe this is because we are not here in this physical existence to amass physical possessions. The proof is in how we feel just a few days or weeks later. Contrast this to how we feel when we find ourselves making a personal difference in the lives of others or when we contribute our time in a philanthropic manner. How does that feel compared to the short-lived joy of the new prize or item? That feeling of making a difference for others stays with you. We don't lose that joy in the same fashion in which we do with the attainment of worldly possessions. That has to mean something when we step back and observe it.

Personally, in my own exploration into the meaning of life, I have chosen to perceive my success within this physical existance with what I have given and served others. I want that type of abundance. I want that form of achievement. Don't misunderstand—I do enjoy this human experience and many of the physical aspects of it. While we are here on Earth , part of the experience is to enjoy our physical existence. We won't be able to enjoy those aspects of life when no longer incarnated (with a physical body). Those experiences, however, just should not become the main avenues through which we label ourselves and our levels of success.

The Authority Label

Many of us live life as we sometimes blindly, yet often faithfully, listen to those in "high places," telling us how we should live our lives. We humans have been groomed to listen and obey. It is true that in order to have a functioning society, we need to have rules, but those who create these rules deserve to be under a watchful eye.

Rules often have good reason for their creation. We stop at red traffic lights and stop signs to avoid causing accidents. It is wise of us to buckle our seat belts before backing the car out of the driveway. Certainly, one would not want to exceed the speed limit by too much lest one receive a speeding ticket. These are just a few of the countless rules that have been created by different authority figures over time. It seems that as our society evolves, we create more rules to help ourselves function in a normal manner. But what happens when we instill too much trust in authority?

In 1963, Stanley Milgram, a psychologist at Yale University, set out to understand just how far people will go when given orders from those with perceived authority. The study began by advertising for males to take part in a study at the university. The first step was to draw lots to decide from the group who would be "learners" and who would be "teachers." The selection was fixed so that the participants were always in a position of being "the teacher," and Milgram's team, pretending to be real participants, always in the position of "learner."

The learner was given the name of Mr. Wallace. Mr. Wallace was hooked up with electrodes on his arms as the teacher watched, and then he was taken into a room. The person playing the part of teacher could not see him but could hear him. The teacher went into a separate room and was shown an electric shock generator that contained a row of switches that read from 15 volts (mild shock) up to 450 volts (dangerous and potentially deadly).

> Fear cannot be our guide, for when we allow it to, it will control and rule us, reciprocating more of the same within our lives keeping us shackled.

In the experiment, the learner, Mr. Wallace, was told to memorize a list of word pairs and their meaning. The teacher then read aloud the word pairs from the other room. Mr. Wallace was expected to describe their meaning. For each incorrect answer, the teacher was told by the authority figure (known as the experimenter) to administer a shock to Mr. Wallace.

Mr. Wallace repeatedly and intentionally gave incorrect answers. The teacher was instructed to provide the corresponding shock with each incorrect answer. If for any reason the teacher didn't administer the appropriate level of shock, he would be reminded by the authority figure to press the correct button to shock Mr. Wallace. There were four responses from the authority figure if the teacher hesitated and didn't provide the shock:

- Please continue.
- The experiment requires that you continue.

- It is absolutely essential that you continue.
- You have no other choice but to continue.

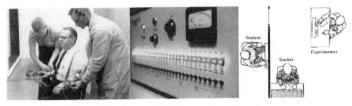

All of this occurred with Mr. Wallace pretending to scream and shout in pain as the fake shocks were administered. He would even get to a point of pleading with the teacher figure, begging them to stop. This study was carried out eighteen times. Sixty-five percent of the time, the teacher went all the way to highest level of 450 volts, capable of causing bodily harm to most people. All the teacher candidates went to at least 300 volts.[6]

Most people are likely to follow orders that they perceive to have been given through a person in authority. Not only were they willing to hurt the individual, but they even went to the full extent of possibly killing an innocent human being. It seems that obedience to those in high positions of authority is ingrained within us all from the very beginning of our programming. We tend to obey orders from others who are identified by their authority. We learn this over time through our families, school systems, governments, and careers.

What would you have done in this situation? We may want to say we would never have participated or would not have gone as far as the teacher candidates did. But in everyday life, humans choose to harm each other when given orders from others in places of perceived power. Look at how many wars were begun in the name of righteousness and propaganda. Who is to say which government leaders are right and which ones are wrong when we kill in the name of democracy? Is not all killing wrong? Yet we as humans see it labeled as OK for certain situations and wrong for others. What would happen if all of us on Earth said,

"No, we shall kill no one else ever again," even if the order for war came from the highest levels of government? What then?

Of course, there is a need for authority in life. But at what point do we begin to question it at higher levels? It is safe to say in many cases we have allowed the authority label to go too far. We sometimes even turn a blind eye to it assuming that it needs to be done in the name of righteousness. Authority itself can even be viewed as a religion, a means through which we respond to fear, for it is through our fears that we allow righteousness. Fear and authority lead us to our next big label in life—religion.

The Religion Label

Have you ever heard of the name Zoroaster? Maybe not, but I'm sure you likely know the names Mohammad, Buddha, and Jesus. The prophet Zoroaster (Zarathrustra in ancient Persian) is regarded as the founder of Zoroastrianism. Zoroaster was a man living in the Bronze Age of Iran nearly 4,000 years ago, and he is credited with the formation of what is believed to have been the world's first monotheistic religion. Zoroastrianism taught that one God, one ruler over all, was responsible for mankind. According to the Zoroastrianism tradition, Zoroaster experienced a divine vision of one supreme God who ruled over everything. He experienced this vision while partaking in a pagan purification rite at the age of thirty. He began teaching followers to worship a single god named Ahura Mazda.

The beliefs of Zoroastrianism were spread through Asia by the use of the Silk Road, a network of trade routes that connected China, the Middle East, and Europe. Some scholars teach and believe that Zoroastrianism helped generate religions such as Judaism, Christianity, and Islam. The power of the Persian Empire at the time bolsters this theory.[7]

The Muslim conquest of Persia during the years of 633—651 AD led to the demise of the Persian Empire and the rejection of Zoroastrianism in Iran. The Arab conquerors began to tax Zoroastrians living in Iran and enacted laws upon them, which made their lives more difficult. The end result was of a drastic shrinking of the following, and most Zoroastrians converted to Islam.[8]

This is just one example of society forcing the views of one group onto another. I believe religion certainly has a place in the world. After all, life without a purpose would be quite a disheartening reality. However, I think many can attest to the fact that while religion can serve for good, it has without question been the proponent of great evil. What a strange paradox. How can something that is born of good generate such hate? It is yet one more issue that requires further exploration.

Perhaps my point of view on this comes from my upbringing. My mother had me baptized as a Catholic when I was a baby. At various times during my youth, I become a member of the Seventh Day Adventist Church, Episcopalian Church, Presbyterian Church, and others. Throughout all of this, I remember each church telling of why they were right on their specific version of the teachings of God.

It made me want to understand at a deeper level why we as humans display a need to tell others what is right and what is wrong. To this day, I will sometimes get people who energetically want to instill in me that their view is right, mine is wrong, and that if I want to be saved, I need to follow and adopt their religion. These are well-meaning individuals who are doing what they believe to be their part, so I don't fault them for trying. However, why can't we simply allow each individual to determine for themselves what they believe to be true? Why the need to force views upon others? We may be more civil than our ancestors about how we go about trying to convert others, but many of us desperately want others to live in the same camp of theory and thought as we do.

It took me a while to get to this point in my personal Ungraduation process and de-labeling. I had to ask myself what the harm was in allowing ourselves and others to discover our own personal religion. This epiphany came through trying to convert my wife to my own views. Shortly after we first met, I found myself asking her about her religious beliefs. I wanted to understand what she thought of life, God, and the afterlife. She would repeatedly tell me her views on religion were that of a "personal connection" with God. When I would push further, I was always met with the same response—that her belief was more personal than anything else. She didn't believe that we had to go to church every Sunday in order to feel God.

I would ask her if she believed she would be saved in life after death if she didn't spend enough time in church and trying to reach a connection with God. She would again respond that she had enough belief in her heart that she and God were just fine and that she didn't feel she needed anything further.

At the time, that was something I just couldn't understand. "But you're supposed to spend time with God at church in order to show him you are a good person," I would reply adamantly. Repeatedly, I would get the same response: "What works for you works for you but doesn't need to be the case for all others." My wife is a wise one indeed and was beyond her years at that time in our lives together.

It wasn't until many years later through my own introspection that I saw she was right. The labels we place on ourselves and others are just ways to fit into society. Our own beliefs and ideas of what comes after death or what the point of life even is should be very personal. One belief doesn't make any other more right or wrong. It is our ever-insistent need to fit ourselves into a box we feel we belong in rather than being the piece of the puzzle that doesn't fit and being quite OK with it. It took me some time, but this is now how I view religious labels—I'm OK being the piece of the puzzle that doesn't quite fit. Especially when it feels more right from a personal perspective rather than being fake just to fit into someone else's life views and labels.

What feels right for you doesn't mean it's right for everyone. We all get to where we need to be when the time is right. We don't need others telling us how we should think, and we certainly don't need religion to be a catalyst for fear—fear of what comes in the afterlife if we don't live a righteous life to the tune of how others tell us is right. But that happens all the time in the last big label of life: politics.

Red vs Blue—The Great Compromise

We may find it hard to envision a more polarizing time than whichever one we are living through. For example, just when we thought it couldn't get any wilder than the 2016 Presidential Campaign, along came the 2020 version. Most Americans and many people across the world found themselves unable to have general thoughts about political matters let alone share those opinions openly.

But perhaps that isn't much different from previous times. The history in the United States is built on the rigorous debate and open dialog of talking through our differences of opinions in an effort to find common ground. It wasn't any different back in 1787, the year the Constitution of the United States was written. As a matter of fact, what our forefathers dealt with may have had even more challenges and ramifications.

During the summer of 1787, eleven years after the colonies declared their independence, we were grappling with how to best run our country. The division was so intense because what was being discussed was how to set up the model that would be used to pass legislation and govern the people. Representatives from small states didn't want to give up the authority they enjoyed under the Articles of the Confederation, and representatives from the states with larger populations felt they should have more standing power. The very topic threatened to end the Constitutional Convention entirely.

It was the well-respected Roger Sherman from Connecticut who made the suggestion to have a proportional representation through a House of Representatives, and a Senate with equal amounts of representation for each state. At the time, the proposition was so radical, it was dismissed quickly by the group. While we are familiar with this way of governing today, it wasn't widely accepted at first. Eventually, what was then known as the Connecticut Compromise became known as the Great Compromise and was adopted. Each side of the political spectrum at the time felt validated in fair representation.[9]

Perhaps it is time to rethink the political labels that have been placed on us. The world is again in need of another Great Compromise. Whether or not we have political leaders decide for us, we can certainly still choose to erase labels from ourselves if we want to. I'm not suggesting that we move out of caring about politics, as I realize operating under political labels is how we currently attempt to tackle large-scale issues in the world. However, there are ways to Ungraduate from the position of seeing ourselves as red, blue, and independent.

First and foremost, we are all human. That is one label that we can all agree on in the political spectrum. We may have our differing views across many controversial topics, but on the whole, one commonality we share is the term given to our species. We are humans first, and then the many labels get placed upon us secondarily.

This is where the Ungraduation process begins in the political arena. Unless you are an individual who is running for an office of local or broader-reaching government, you likely don't need to classify yourself in any one bucket of the political spectrum. Yes, we know that some of our views may align with different aspects of the political label umbrellas, but we can choose to free ourselves from classifying ourselves as under those umbrellas.

For example, I was born into a Democrat family. We were classified as poor, and at the time, I believe my mother aligned more with the want to be supported through the government. Perhaps not that she wanted to, but we certainly needed it then. We were on welfare and food stamps at the time as my mother struggled to make ends meet as a single mother of two children.

As I grew up, I stayed mostly underneath the Democrat label. I began to form my own opinions and investigated which party more aligned with my views. At the time, I was very much looking to fit within a label to define me and my views. I switched to the Republican Party label in my mid to late twenties.

Time went on, and I continued to watch the political spectrum. It became apparent to me that I didn't align or fall into either side—not even close. As I did some research, I found that even the Independent and Libertarian parties each had a certain belief.

In my own search to separate from the identity of political labels, I wrote my state and asked that moving forward, they completely remove my party affiliation for me. I no longer wanted to be classified as a Democrat or a Republican. I also wasn't going to choose to call myself an Independent or a Libertarian. I simply wanted the label No Party. Now, whether or not the state honored my request, I'm not sure. But I followed the instructions of my state to put in that specific request. I see myself as *human* and do not want any political label attached to my name. Mostly because none of them completely identifies me. Nor will they likely completely align with your views. I can still vote, still take part in political conversations, and certainly contribute to my constitutional duties as I see fit, but I now do so from a freeing mindset of not being labeled as being inside of one party or another.

I want to see people for who they are—human first. In today's completely politically polarized world, how freeing it is to say, "I am affiliated with no party." That isn't to say we should be turning a blind eye to the political landscape, just simply that we are not defined by the labels by which others will identify us.

Moreover, it is my personal belief that the modern political system has really become "two wings of the same bird." The more

I look at the political world, the more it appears to blend together. The same issues will likely continue to crop up and generate debate, and those same issues will likely continue to be problematic well into the future.

Political views and agendas are always changing. Some topics and beliefs will remain largely under the "red" or "blue" umbrella, while there will be many topics that find unified agreement from both sides. No matter the outcome of these debates, the one great compromise that I think would benefit us all is to see each other as human first and without all the labels we try to place on ourselves and each other.

Ungraduated Call to Action:

- What are some labels that you are putting on others that are keeping you from having deeper understandings and relationships with the people?
- What labels are you using to "define" yourself in regard to authority, religion, and politics? While these all may play important roles in your life, they are not you. Work to "wear" your labels but not become them.
- What compromises have you made that could be holding you back in your life regarding your own labels or the labels you have given others?

Chapter 3

Seeing the Laws, Obeying the Laws

"There is nothing more deceptive than an obvious fact."
~ Sir Arthur Conan Doyle ~

Heading to Singapore soon? If so, leave the gum at home. It's illegal there for the simple fact that it cost mass transit and housing development communities $150,000 annually to remove it from sidewalks and surfaces. Chewing gum, with the exception of nicotine and therapeutic varieties, is illegal and includes fines and jail time for anyone caught possessing it.

I hope that if you find yourself traveling on the autobahn in Germany, you are properly fueled up. If not, running out of gas on that superhighway will result in a fine. And if you do run out of gas, don't think of walking to a gas station because that will levy you another fine—it's all about safety concerns. The Germans believe that people using the autobahn have a responsibility to check their fuel levels before getting on to travel. Failure to keep your car fueled well enough to make the complete trip will not only damage your ego but also leave a dent in your wallet.

Apparently, my wife and I bucked the system in Venice, Italy, where it is illegal to feed the pigeons. In 2008, lawmakers officially made it illegal

> Universal Law is not subjective as in Man's Law. Under Universal Law, the definition of what is "right" and "wrong" is the same for everyone, everywhere.

to feed the pesky birds due to the cleanup efforts they make necessary in St. Mark's Square. It was reportedly costing each citizen €275 annually to take care of the mess. That being unbeknownst to us, we fed them anyway on a summer trip there in 2018. We were standing in St. Mark's Square holding food on outstretched hands as the birds landed on our arms to graze from whatever it was that we were holding. Had we gotten caught, we could have faced fines up to €700. My wife and I escaped with photos of her feeding the birds, no worse for wear. I guess we could have claimed ignorance, which would have been true, but I'm thankful we didn't have to explain ourselves to the Italian authorities.

These are just a smattering of some of the odd and unusual laws laid out around the world. Each of them likely serves a purpose to some extent, even though they may seem strange. The one commonality of most laws is that they are created by humans with the hope that they better serve the masses.

As a society, we function mostly within rules that have been laid out for us by other people or governments. These laws change over time as society and leaders deem fit. For example, it was once fine to drink alcohol before we made it illegal during the years of Prohibition in the early twentieth century. We then overturned that law and once again deem it acceptable to drink alcohol. Whether illegal or not and despite what the law stated at the time, people still decided to consume alcohol if they felt the desire and could obtain it.

The examples above can pertain to many different aspects of manmade law. We decide what is acceptable or unacceptable. This does not, however, work within the laws of the Universe. These rules are finite. Whether we accept them, believe in them, like or dislike them, they exist and cannot be changed. I implore you not to be the individual who decides to test these Universal Laws as you aim to defy gravity walking off a cliff expecting not plunge to your death. The key to this understanding is to learn how to operate and maximize the Universal Laws we are bound by while in this physical reality we call life and live in harmony alongside them.

There are seven Universal Laws that deserve more understanding in regard to how the Universal Field of energy works. While some of these Universal Laws can be debated, it is my experience that they are very much real. We stand to benefit by a great degree if we can operate within these laws. However, the penalties of not realizing these laws exist are far greater than any monetary fines that we could get from our own government and legal authorities.

Universal Law
Principle 1—Mentalism

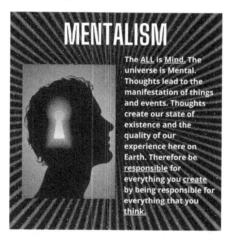

Where did the phrase "mind over matter" come from? Likely, many people have heard that phrase at one point or another. Typically, it is when we are engaged in some sort of struggle or challenge. Perhaps we are engaged in a strenuous physical activity, or feverishly working toward a future goal. Why would such a saying exist, and where did it come from?

In the *Kybalion*, it is stated, "The All is Mind; the Universe is mental." The ancient Hermetic book goes onto explain that The All is the substantial reality underlying all the outward manifestations and appearances that we know under the terms of the Universe. This of course includes the physical and nonphysical aspects of matter and energy. In short, all that is apparent to our material senses is Spirt, which in itself may be considered and thought of as a universal, infinite, living mind.

> Be mindful of your thoughts and self-talk—you are literally thinking your life into existence each moment of every day.

Now that is a lot to wrap your mind around—literally. The suggestion is that the Universe was generated by the mind of the Creator, and that all things experienced within our known Universe exist within this mind, as we are one and a part of it. This certainly ties into the teachings of the Bible as well: "In the beginning, God created the Heavens and the Earth ." Could that famous line of scripture from the Bible really mean the physical, which we see, Earth and Universe, along with the nonphysical, which we do not see? Could Heaven be an allegorical reference to the nonphysical reality?

The principle of mentalism aligns very closely to the book of Genesis in the Old Testament of the Bible outlining the creation of the "Heavens and the Earth ." The *Kybalion* explains the true nature of energy, power, and form along with how all of these are subordinate to the mastery of Mind.

Therefore, it is so important to be mindful of our thoughts. Seeking to become aware that what we think, on every level, is a manifestation—a potentiality that can be brought into our physical existence. Thought exists on the mental plane (heavenly plane if you wish to see it that way), and we manifest our thoughts into our physical planes where we exist every day. Whatever we think most about grows and materializes in our lives.

Our entire physical existence could very well be our training grounds for when we are without a physical body and then are only of conscious thought energy (spirit). Keep mindful of your thoughts because you likely are thinking things into existence one thought at a time. They may not come into existence overnight, but be very certain that over a period of weeks, months, and years, we do absolutely morph into a culmination of our daily thoughts, for better or for worse.

Universal Law Principle 2— Correspondence

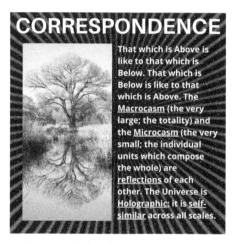

"As above so below, and as below so above; as within, so without; as without, so within."

The second principled law of the Universe embodies the truth that there will always be a correspondence between the laws and natural phenomenon that occur between the various planes of existence in which the Universe operates. Coming to this realization is what can allow an individual to examine solutions to problems that exist above and below surface level. What is meant by this is having the ability to truly analyze a problem's real point of manifestation.

For example, if an individual is dealing with a dilemma concerning lack of self-confidence, the problem can be analyzed through different lenses. There are many different aspects to this, but we will look at a few possible angles of how the principle applies.

A person dealing with a confidence issue is dwelling on situations in their past that have been brought into the present moment. The problem may have originated with one example, or even several examples from the past in which this person failed in some regard. It may even have been perpetuated by other people taunting and antagonizing the person at that moment in the past.

Because we only truly live and operate within the *present moment*, constantly dwelling on a lack of self-confidence continues to materialize within the everyday present moment. This constant dwelling on a lack of confidence is being brought in from the realm of thought (a different plane of existence from what we see with our physical eyes), and manifesting in the present moment. The plane, or realm, of thought is not bound by time. It happens always in the now.

> Time doesn't actually exist. What issues are you corresponding with from your past that are hindering you "now" in the ever-present moment?

Humans invented the concept of time for our need to function. However, in a larger sense, time does not actually exist. If you were to ask a bird what time it is (assuming we could ever converse with any species on Earth other than our own) the bird would likely respond, "The time is now." Now is the only time it ever really is. Time is a manmade fabrication, as we only truly ever live in *the now*—the past was at one time lived, and the future will be lived in present moments as well. We never physically operate in the past or the future, but we bring the thought of those times into our current state. The solution to this problem is simply to change the mindset and stop focusing on the moments in the past or worry of the future. It's necessary to live in the now.

This is just one example of how to understand and use the principle of correspondence. Many of our current problems are simply aspects of our daily thoughts. I know it sounds easier to say than to do, but we literally can change our lives for the better by being able to properly analyze our thought activities. By making it a practice to observe our own thoughts, we gain the ability to become mindful. Becoming mindful then puts us more in touch with the present moment, which then shapes our future, one day at a time—hopefully for the better.

This is how we get life to "correspond" with us and for us. As the French philosopher René Descartes famously first said, "I think, therefore I am." This principle is absolute. It works for the positive and the negative. Think positively. and you will bring in more positive aspects; think negatively, and you'll certainly attract more negativity into your life. This equates to cause and effect, which we will address shortly.

Universal Law Principle 3—Vibration

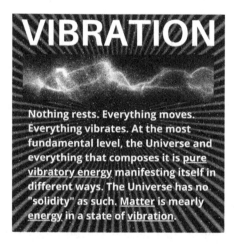

Everything in life is vibrating. Everything is made up of energy. The chair I sit on as I type is not actually solid. It is made up of billions and billions of tiny atoms swirling around at such a fast pace that the chair appears solid and even holds me in place. But the chair is not actually solid. It is vibrating at inconceivable speed to hold together and "appear solid." Science and physics have come a long way over the centuries, and in the modern era, we have come to understand energy is at the center of everything. We have become even more enlightened recently that atoms are actually empty space.

Here are some mind-bending statistics—an atom's nucleus is only a few femtometers across. A femtometer is a word. I didn't just make it up, though it sounds like it. A femtometer is about a thousand million millionth of a meter. Super, super, super incredibly small. So now we need to understand exactly how far away the electrons are from the nucleus of the atom. They travel around the nucleus at a distance of one-ten-billionth of a meter away from the core. To right size this—it's 100,000 times the width of the nucleus. A comparison to this would be if the nucleus were a basketball centered in Manhattan, then the electrons flying around it would be circling from about the distance from the basketball to Philadelphia. All the space in between the rotation is *empty space*.

So back to the start of all this, the chair I'm sitting on right now is really made up of empty space. I know it sounds crazy, but it's now a scientifically proven truth. The electrons and the nuclei are constantly engaging through the force known as electromagnetism. Each circumference around the atom is carried about the rotation through an electronic force of a particle of pure energy called a proton. Each proton pushes back with equal force, a tiny push or pull enabled across the emptiness in space. That, along with some other quantum physics jargon, is really what's keeping my butt from drifting through the stuff I call my chair. It is really all the energy force of this process that holds the chair together.[10]

Enough with the science lesson. I loved science in high school. It was one subject I was really interested in and did well with, but it is not for everyone. What you just need to understand is that *everything* we see in the physical world is made up of energy. This energy is in constant vibration and movement. Even the human body vibrates with energy. The body can generate mechanical vibrations at very low frequencies, so-called infrasonic waves. Different organs of the human body produce different resonance frequencies. For example, the heart resonance frequency vibrates at 1 hertz. The brain has a resonance frequency of 10 hertz.

Everything we see in life is vibrating at a set pace; some quickly and some really slowly. To understand this, think of a tire on a car or truck moving *very* fast. It can almost appear that it is not moving at all, right? At the lowest levels of vibration, objects move extremely slowly. So slowly, they appear to be not moving at all. Think rocks and trees. Between these two states of super fast and very slow, there exist infinite manifestations all occurring at varying octaves of vibration, each with their own existence and reactionary states.

Human thought has its own certain level of vibration and can be controlled, like tuning an instrument to produce differing results.

> You do not attract into your life what you desire; you attract into life what you actually are. Your vibration is you.

We can aim to generate self-improvement in this physical form and perhaps even manifest thoughts into existence in our own lives. As we can better understand vibration—our own frequency, harmony, and resonance increase, and we gain more power over ourselves and our world, individually and collectively. This is the way that we ultimately can control and better ourselves, along with the entire world.[11]

Universal Law Principle 4—Polarity

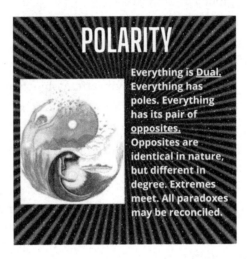

Opposites attract. Certainly, that's a rule I have seen alive and well in my life. My life partner, my wife, is my opposite in almost every way. She balances me by countering my opinion when I need a different perspective. She and I think differently, yet also appreciate each other's points of view. Polarity is what has made our marriage unique and at times quite entertaining. This fourth principle contains the truth that everything has its opposite, and that all things have two poles existing in a state of constant duality. The secret behind this principle is that opposites are really *the same*, only varying by small degrees in difference. Opposites are simply extremes of the same thing. An example of this is hot and cold. Both are simply a description of temperature, varying only in degree. There is no clear-cut point when hot stops being hot, and cold starts being cold. When is hot actually hot? Is it at 80° (27° Celsius)? Maybe 85° (29° Celsius)? 95° (35° Celsius)?

> Life gives us the test each day to work on improving our practice of mental alchemy. Take notice of the differing degrees of emotions within you as you live each day.

The same goes for light and darkness, hard and soft, big and small, even love and hate. With love and hate, there is no clear point where one emotion becomes another or when it passes through like, dislike, or indifference. All these examples are left up to individual perceptions of the degree. The principle of Polarity exists to explain these paradoxes.

This principle is important because it implies that we can adjust the polarity of a degree of emotion by recognizing it is the same emotion, and choosing the degree that best suits our needs. We often experience involuntary and rapid transitions in our psyche between love and hate, like and dislike, as well as various other emotions. Ultimately, our goal should be to notice these emotions as we experience them and choose to experience these transitions through the use of our willpower for the betterment of our life and the lives of others. The better we get at recognizing emotions and feelings within us, the more we are brought into a more present moment of existence. Recognizing the differences of extremes is not an insurmountable challenge. They are simply expressions of the same thing differing by degrees.

This practice of recognizing and adjusting to these polarities can be known or described as the art of Mental Alchemy. *The Alchemist*, by Paulo Coelho, a short easy read, speaks to a great story of a man on a journey to find his purpose, thinking it is externally located in Egypt. All the while he possesses it within, and ultimately discovers the way to his purpose through his mind and awareness. We each have a daily opportunity to work on mastering this art. We must awaken to truth and realize that the potential to discover real treasures is within us. It takes time and commitment. Treasure chests full of rewards are not typically lying out in the open for easy taking. We must dig deep and work to find them.

Universal Law Principle 5—Rhythm

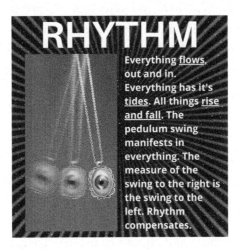

We have all felt emotional highs and lows. We love staying in the highs of life and always want to get out of the lows as quickly as possible. The phrase, "this too shall pass" was created to be ever in view and is true and appropriate in all times and situations. The legend goes that an Eastern monarch had asked his speech writers to come up with a phrase that could always be used in all ever-present moments. They presented him the words: "And this, too, shall pass away." Abraham Lincoln employed these words in this speech as well just before his inauguration as he became the 16th president of the United States. The words are evergreen and present for a reason of truth.[12] Existing between the extremes of Polarity is the pendulum swing of Rhythm. This principle embodies the fact that everything exists in measured motion. Here to there, in and out, backward and forward, the rise and fall; everything always moving and flowing and never truly being still. The Universe is always flowing, never stopping, and always changing. This principle points to the cycle of life and death, creation and destruction, rise and fall, and of course manifests within us as we experience different forms of emotions and mental states. When we understand this, we can use it to our advantage by polarizing ourselves to the degrees we desire. Meaning we can *choose* to be happy, or we can literally choose ourselves negative daily. Now, when positive and negative things happen to us, we can also choose how to respond to those things, knowing that they are not going to last. Bringing awareness to these life transitions can be the difference between weeks, months, and years of recovery (mentally, physically, and emotionally), or short, intermittent grace periods between times of intensity. These are aspects of knowing thyself and trying to work toward emotional mastery.

With a heightened level of awareness around the principle of Rhythm, we can experience transcendental states of consciousness to enable ourselves to stay above the swing of the pendulum. Rhythm is always going to have an effect on us one way or another. However, being in control will help guide us forward and bring us back into accountability and control of ourselves.

> Rather than being the pendulum swing, become the observer of the pendulum swings of your life.
> It's far easier to weather the highs and lows.

People who experience self-mastery do this to some degree, but those who intently focus their will upon this principle are able to act from a place of purpose as opposed to allowing the emotions, or proverbial swing of the pendulum, to take them for a ride. It certainly helps to understand that we have a choice when it comes to our observations and responses in life. The key is never allowing ourselves to get too high or too low when life happens.

The game of life is going to take us on twists and turns and up mountains and down into valleys. We just need to stay aware that we do have some ability to control the accelerator as well as to let off the brakes when we need to. Buckle up and realize that there are no one-way streets in this game. We must always play as active participants for the best chance of coming out on top in the end.

Universal Law Principle 6— Cause & Effect

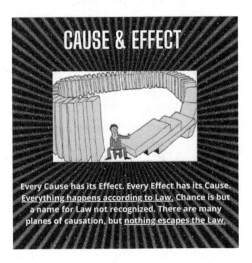

I think this is my favorite principle. It's the one I wish more of humanity could understand. In order to create change, we must begin with us. Too often, people do one of two things. They get angry with the world and decide to become belligerent and outrageous, yelling, protesting, becoming angry with what they see around them; or they become a recluse and retreat to their own realities, putting blinders up and pretending the outside world does not exist.

The third type of people make up a much smaller group. They are the ones who understand on an individual and collective level that real change occurs from our individual and collective thought. In order to bring about change in our lives, we must create it ourselves. Being upset, complaining about the world's problems, and becoming negative does nothing but result in more of those things. Standing by idly does not work either. We individually and collectively bring into our physical world what we think. This is cause and effect.

This principle means nothing ever happens by chance. There is a reason for everything. Every decision we make has an outcome. This principle is in harmony with the principle of Correspondence. There are higher planes of existence that dominate the lower planes, and all throughout these planes of existence, nothing escapes the Principle of Cause & Effect. Everything comes with explanation if we really examine it.

The way to use this principle with more empowerment is to consciously become aware of how it works. Be aware and *watch* your thoughts. Realize that the mental plane (plane of thought) is where we spend a great deal of time. Become *mindful* of thought. Become the catalyst for your life.

Through our thoughts, we are literally thinking our lives into existence. Think in an anxious and fearful manner, and you will bring more of those emotions into your life. Think in a calm and peaceful way, and you will have more abundance of those types of reactions in life.

We can put into action the first move, which will bring us the result we desire, not as a surprise but a product of calculation. Can we see how this relates to the principle of Correspondence?

We often say we want to live better lives and become better leaders and individuals. Well, what steps does that entail? Perhaps we choose to focus on writing each day and reading more often as opposed to not doing those things and finding the excuses to sit around and watch more television and news. When we do not do the work required, we resign to merely reacting to the consequences of not having put in the time. We experience the problems that inevitably come when we are not pursuing our highest calling.

> Become the cayalyst for your life—how you think generates how you act, and how you act dictates your outcomes in life. Nothing escapes cause and effect.

Without fail, when you are on a quest to become

a person who has mastery over him- or herself and have better control of your feelings, personality, and environment, you will naturally be in unison with the higher planes in accordance to this principle. When one becomes more aware of this Universal Law of cause and effect, it is impossible to act out of alignment with higher principles. Having awareness of this will give you the ability to take control on the physical plane of existence without walking through life in utter disarray and lack of control.

We are individually and collectively creating our own worlds. We can choose to ignore what we see, hoping that someone else will come along and change it. We can get upset and scream and yell at the people doing what we don't like, or we can all look within and become better at controlling our mental thoughts and manifesting what we want here in the physical world. We do not need help from any external force to set us free. We have that power within ourselves.

Universal Law Principle 7—Gender

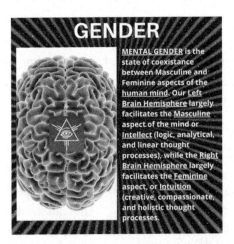

Masculinity and femininity are found in all aspects of life. This does not simply apply just in sex, as male and female. It applies to the way that nature is created and in the creative aspects of all things on Earth and on all other planes of existence. Once again, this principle also ties back to the second principle of Correspondence. Masculinity and femininity exist in the physical plane, the mental (thought plane), and the spiritual plane as well. Gender plays a role in all things from generation, creation, and regeneration. Literally existence cannot come into being without this principle.

The masculine side of Gender is the more aggressive, conquest driven, explorative energy that drives progress. The feminine is the openminded, sacred, treasured, protective energy that maintains tradition and honors the priority of what is most important, while nourishing and maintaining that which is most essential to life.

This also materializes in the left-brain versus right-brain aspects of thought. You may have heard of the characteristics of left-brain people being more critical in thought, practicality, and immersed in the details of life. Little can be true for these thinkers unless proven through factual evidence. Then there are the those who are right-brain thinkers who express themselves in the arts, are more receptive to new perspectives, and tend to be more creative and open in their thinking. Left-brain tends to be more masculine based, and right-brain can be seen as more feminine. The key is to try to balance this thinking in order to become the most aware and effective in our everyday lives.

> Choose the middle path of balance between emotions and critical thinking. We need both in order to achieve our greatest outcomes in life.

Too much masculine energy, without a good balance of feminine, can lead to a power struggle to the extremes of possible reckless abandon. In this modality, we lose perspective on what is most important and forget the principles that began our purpose in the first place. Masculine energy tends to be forward and future based. Too much feminine energy, without a balance of the masculine, can leave people dangling without action, purpose, and causation—too lost in their own thoughts. Feminine energy tends to remain in the present moment and does not lean too far into the future.

All beings contain this Gender principle. They exist as two parts for the whole. Every male has feminine energy, and every female has masculine energy. In some, the scales tip far to the extremes. The goal again is to get the best return and insight to balance ourselves as we use both these energies to their fullest extent.

The most exponential use of this principle is how Gender can be made responsible for creation, generation, and regeneration on the mental and spiritual planes, and not just the physical plane of existence. Power can truly be found through the balancing of the Gender energies within us regarding our relationships and environments.

By tuning in to these energies, we can begin to realize truths regarding how present we are with our lives, how focused we are on the future, and what we have sacrificed for our goals and aspirations. We can choose to protect and honor our highest priorities. We can see how far we have stretched our learning and development in pursuit of what we desire most. Lastly, we see how much we are willing to give in order to receive.

This is how we evaluate internally if these energies are in balance. Choosing the middle path between these extremes and seeking balance in all things is one of the keys to becoming centered regarding how to best achieve what we want out of life.

Breaking the Shackles of Critical Thinking

Critical thinking is necessary for advancement in life. But often, we limit ourselves through our unwillingness to be uncomfortable with what cannot be tangibly explained. Albert Einstein was one of the greatest thinkers of all time. But he was so caught up in logic that he often couldn't see what was right in front of him.

As the father of modern physics, Einstein didn't like quantum mechanics. Much of his work stands as the foundation that helped build quantum mechanics, but there were some aspects of quantum mechanics that didn't sit well with him. Einstein didn't like the probability aspects. He preferred something that was much more deterministic and finite.

Referring to the discovery of the Higgs Boson particle from chapter one, Einstein dubbed this type of result "Spooky action at a distance." He couldn't understand it. It wasn't tangible enough to him and didn't sit well on his mind. How could it be that one particle at one place in time could respond exactly like another particle miles away?[13]

What he was missing was the connected understanding that scientists are now beginning to discover. We do live within and operate under a Universal Law that impacts our lives in deeply profound ways. These Universal Laws often get chalked up to *coincidence*. As stated earlier, this raises the question: "How many coincidences can we add up before they become mathematically improbable?" We all contain atoms and particles. Our thought energy is constantly stimulating them. That energy impacts us and our good luck or misfortune as well as the lives of others.

We may believe that laws come from those who have the best view from their position of high command and authority. The view is far better for us if we begin to climb all the way to the top and over those who create temporary and changing rules and regulations. Manmade law is important to understand. It is imperative that we gain understanding of Universal Laws so we can live our lives with the most harmony possible. These are the real laws that we need to begin to see, understand, and obey.

Ungraduated Call to Action

- When can you remember some specific examples in your life that you experienced any of the seven principles of Universal Laws? What are they, and what were the outcomes?

- List out some "strange coincidences" that you recall happening in your life—could these be tied back to any of the seven principles of Universal Law? If so, which ones?
- What were any "synchronicities" that have occurred in your life? Can you begin seeing their meaning?

Part 2
Personal Abundance & Growth

Chapter 4
The Thirst for Knowledge

"Knowing yourself is the beginning of all Wisdom."
~Aristotle~

Picture you are living in the Middle Ages. Some at this time believed the Earth to be flat. It certainly appears that way from all physical aspects of perception. No one had flown in an airplane, let alone been to outer space to challenge the common belief. Would you have simply accepted it to be so since others told you this was the case? Or would your frame of perspective allow your mind to consider any other possibility?

There is a vast difference between learning through self-discovery and being told through another perspective how to think about certain topics. Certainly, this does not apply to all categories; mathematics is rather black and white and only works one way. We can choose to believe that 1+1=3, but in reality, it will always equal two. However, when it comes to history, biology, and even modern science, there is much that is changing. What you or I may have been taught in the education system may not actually align with complete truths.

Knowledge, particularly self-knowledge, is what generates freedom of thought. As we question and find out more about the origin of our history, we sometimes find more questions than answers. Many of the answers we are finding don't align with current teachings. This results in some topics that

> A closed mind will never advance, for the minds of those that believe they are always right believe they have nothing left to learn.

are fiercely debated. We are talking about the possibility of needing to rewrite history books. One can probably understand the reason for such hesitancy, but if the facts are aligning and proving points of variation, then further exploration and questioning are warranted. Should this be so surprising?

I was in school twenty-something years ago. Why should I expect the exact same teaching to be applied today? Education is not a onetime affair. Situations and perspectives change. New learnings and discoveries occur. This sometimes happens at a rapid pace, and it should be understood that new discoveries sometimes fight uphill battles. There is a lot of ego and determination that can limit the communication of new discoveries. Entire theories and practical understanding have been built atop the teachings that have been handed down from generation to generation. It is understandable that new learnings and discoveries can face criticism trying to get into the mainstream network of communication. The human ego doesn't often take kindly to being wrong. For that reason, we deserve to continue to ask and seek the answers to form our own truths and understanding.

Reexamining Our History

During my days in the education system, I was taught something I am sure many can relate to. I was taught that civilization has been around for about 5,000 years, and modern-day humans are the most advanced version ever to walk the earth.

Most modern-day education systems teach that between 5,000 and 5,500 years ago, the ancient Sumerians existed along with ancient Egyptians. We know of the Mayan, Incan, Greek, and Roman Empires reigning throughout the past 5,000 years as well. But were these the only major empires and civilizations of humankind?

Modern evidence is beginning to suggest otherwise. Quite frankly, if we really ponder the thought, we should ask ourselves this: What is the likelihood that our planet has been around for nearly 4.5 billion years with civilization only existing for 5,000 of those years? That is such a minuscule amount of time compared to the overall point of reference. My own learning and self-discovery as an adult led me to evidence that there have been civilizations existing much further back in time and that these civilizations likely were just as technologically advanced as we are today—if not more so.

Caral, Peru is just one such example that has shaken historians to their core. Archaeologists and historians alike have been excavating the location in Peru that is proving to have been in existence some 5,000–7,000 years ago and collapsing around the time that we have been taught civilization began.

Previously it had been thought to be around 5,000 years old, but archeologists are uncovering artifacts that predate that 5,000-year mark. Evidence is surfacing that shows advanced civilizations existed 2,000 years earlier than what modern history books have been teaching regarding the beginnings of human civilization.

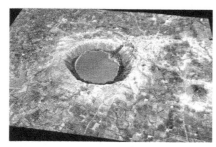

The evidence uncovered about Caral shows they understood geometry and astronomy as shown in some of the discoveries archaeologists have uncovered within the 150-acre site where Caral used to exist.

The new discovery of Caral is not the only situation proving that highly intelligent human civilizations have existed even further back in time. Another technologically advanced civilization existed within modern-day southern Turkey, known as Gobekli Tepe.

Some modern-day historians and scientists have been constrained within their programming or perceived education. They have refused to accept the results of the testing of the pottery extracted from the geological excavations in Gobekli Tepe.

This goes to show the limitations we can place on ourselves by keeping our minds closed and closely aligned to only one perceived reality. When hard and true evidence is placed in front of us, we have the possibility to look right through it or label it as "impossible" or even "conspiracy" since it does not fit our narrative or that of the commonly believed theory.

Fortunately, there are some who persist beyond their beliefs and open their minds to new possibilities and outcomes. That is precisely what German scientist Klaus Schmidt did in the 1990s as he went to Gobekli Tepe to study and date the findings. (For more information see Greg Braden's *Missing Links: The Anomalous History of Humanity*, produced by Gaia.)

It has been discovered through using earth-penetrating radar that Gobekli Tepe consists of five to eight buried circular temples of vertical columns. Because the artifacts have been buried underground for so many years, they have been preserved in a pristine manner. In looking through the artifacts, scientists are finding that this culture had knowledge of constellations and star systems that we thought had not been discovered until the twentieth century.

So how old is Gobekli Tepe? The evidence is suggesting that it dates back between 11,300 and 11,500 years ago. So, now we are at a point where we have more than doubled the previously taught and believed oldest technologically advanced civilizations on earth.[14]

Then there are sites such as Mohenjo-Daro and Harappa, located between present-day Pakistan and India. Archeologists are uncovering artifacts that show these civilizations had indoor plumbing, electricity via underground conduits, stained-glass windows, and batteries. These technologically advanced societies had mathematics and technologies that we have today.

However, a more ominous tale is being unearthed from these historic locations. Archeologists are finding human skeletal remains in "postures of flight," meaning they were fleeing something. They have been found huddled together in families and even with their pets. What is odd about these discoveries is that the remains are being tested and found to have much higher amounts of radiation than they should from simply resting in the earth. The same has been found from clay pots and other artifacts that have been found *vitrified*, meaning they were exposed to such extreme heat that the minerals melted. To cause vitrification, heat must have a rapid onset and extreme intensity.

The Hindu Mahabharata teachings, specifically the Bhagavad Gita portion of these ancient teachings, tells a story of two armies that were engaged in war. One side was losing and resorted to using an unthinkable weapon that inflicted massive and catastrophic damage. Below are some excerpts from the Ancient Mahabharata that describes the event:

> A single projectile charged with all the power of the Universe. An incandescent column of smoke and flame as bright as a thousand suns rose in all its splendor...
>
> A perpendicular explosion with its billowing smoke clouds ... the cloud of smoke rising after its first explosion formed into expanding round circles like the opening of giant parasols...
>
> It was an unknown weapon, an iron thunderbolt, a gigantic messenger of death, which reduced to ashes the entire race of the Vrishnis and the Andhakas.... The corpses were so burned as to be unrecognizable. The hair and nails fell out; Pottery broke without apparent cause, and the birds turned white. After a few hours, all foodstuffs were infected.... To escape from this fire, the soldiers threw themselves in streams to wash themselves and their equipment.[15]

Before the twentieth century, this story had been thought to have been fantasy. However, now we can see the comparisons drawn between what happened to this ancient civilization and that of Hiroshima and Nagasaki Japan on August 6, 1945. The history books are written to tell a story that the United States was the only nation to use an atomic weapon. Perhaps the United States was the only nation in modern times but not the only civilization to ever have used an atomic weapon.

Google Earth has photographic evidence of a large crater positioned in the ground near where these described events took place. Scientists excavated the site to see if the crater was created by an asteroid, but upon digging to the bottom, they found no evidence of any such event. This generates more merit to the validity of the story from the Bhagavad Gita.

Obviously, these examples stir up quite a bit of controversy, but that is precisely what they should do. If an atomic weapon of sorts had been used 5,000 years ago in Mohenjo-Daro, then it would paint a vastly different portrait of the history of mankind.

Are we simply choosing to ignore the evidence because it does not align with what we have been taught? Do we turn a blind eye to this because we do not want to believe we are not the only technologically advanced society to walk the earth?

Perhaps we should lean in and take a closer look and do our research rather than accepting what others have downloaded into our mental program. We should be ever curious and not take what we are taught to perceive at face value without our own confirmed stamp of approval. If we look hard enough, we will see that science is painting a different perspective of our history.

We can trace back and see the cycles of time of where civilization has risen and fallen. It is becoming ever clearer that we are not the only advanced society to walk the earth. What can we learn from previous civilizations that may help us be better in the present?

What we know changes as new discoveries are made. Some historians and scientists are hesitant to share this newfound knowledge as it possibly could threaten history as we've all been made to believe it to be. It is part of the Ungraduation process to look at everything with keen interest and curiosity. Our history books should be no different. I was once taught that Pluto was a planet. Then it was not, then it was again . . . What else will we find out to be true if we continue to intuitively question, poke, prod, and seek more understanding?

Lifelong Learning

Many have the false perception that learning stops once schooling ends. However, education only ends when we choose to end it. No matter what level of education we have completed, weaving continued learning into our lifestyle has positive benefits for personal growth and truth-seeking. Sometimes it is necessary to Ungraduate and relearn aspects of our past education.

It has been said that knowledge is power, but knowledge is only power when acted upon. In order to take correct action on the knowledge we have been given, we must do our part to investigate and get the entire view. For it is within this empowerment seeing and learning for ourselves that we will find our truth to our action and purpose.

One of the best cases of lifelong learning and its practicality is the life of Nelson Mandela. His autobiography, *Long Walk to Freedom*, was written almost exclusively from his position of a lifelong learner. Dr. Peter Rule, a researcher dedicated to the study and research of Mandela's life, drew insights from Mandela as a lifelong learner. Rule described Mandela as having a "very specific emphasis on learning" when he would meet new people, whether they were his friends or enemies. Mandela's autobiography, biographies, and speeches given by and about him reflect these characteristics.

Mandela attributed much of the foundation of his basic education on his Thembu Tribe upbringing. "I was groomed, like my father before me, to counsel the leaders of the tribe." He was educated about his people and culture of the Thembu people, their folklore and law, along with their history. When his father died, Nelson became part of the chief's compound and was able to experience in a personal way what was being decided on in his community. That helped him craft his leadership style.

Nelson Mandela's formal education was diverse. He attained his bachelor's degree at the University of South Africa and a high-level law degree at the University of Witwatersrand. Rule states, "His university education was probably not as significant as we think university education is. But of particular importance for Mandela was the people he met. At Wits, he met lawyers from other racial and cultural backgrounds, and interacted with them at a political and professional level, and that was powerfully formative for him."

> Studies show that people who engage in lifelong learning are happier, healthier, and have more of a zest for life.

He met a variety of people with diverse backgrounds, and he interacted with them on a personal and professional level. He described this as extremely influential in his life.

When he spent time in jail for opposing his country's government, he received education there as well. He was forced to make a life behind bars at Robben Island for twenty-seven years that was described by Mandela himself as "struggle university." "Prisoners created their own curriculum, both academic and political. You could choose to go to class on Marxism, or the Indian struggle, trade unions, or English literature. People who knew about these things would teach," said Rule.

In trying to find the common threads of lifelong learning for Mandela, Rule found what he describes as four levels of dialog:

- With others
- With self
- With the collective
- With context

Mandela refused to dehumanize his adversaries, a.k.a. the other. "He insisted on seeing 'the other' as a person he could acknowledge, understand, interact with, and learn from," states Rule. In his dialog with "the self," he was always searching for more understanding and self-reflection in moments of intense transformative personal learning. Mandela's conversation with the collective shows up in one example of his time interacting with the former liberation, now-ruling party of the African National Congress, or ANC. Lastly in regard to context, Mandela exemplified this dialog and learning when he was released from prison and had to adapt to a new and very different South Africa. It had become violent and was in the midst of transitions of power that he quickly had to understand and adapt to.[16]

So, we can see that Mandela was astute in his understanding of the need to constantly be evolving in his learning and thinking. Not only did he make lifelong learning a passion, he also didn't allow any situation to deter him from learning more. Even his twenty-seven years behind bars didn't stop him from continuing to develop and rethink his points of views. His Ungraduation of learning and relearning new perspectives and rethinking was prevalent throughout his life, and it prepared him for some of life's great experiences.

While many of us won't be able to reach the status and level of impact that Nelson Mandela achieved in his lifetime, why should we approach lifelong learning any differently? We have the opportunity each day to approach life with new and fresh perspectives. What we have been taught in the past need not become cemented and unchangeable in our minds. Quite the opposite. We should approach life with curiosity and ask more questions about what we have been taught. New discoveries and learnings are leading to an everchanging landscape that will likely continue to look different for us in the coming years and decades.

Do we want to stay rigid in the belief systems that have been handed down to us, or do we want to continue to seek out new possibilities that will free our thinking and lead us to new possibilities and results? The Ungraduation process can lead us to some shocking discoveries, but that is what the thirst for more knowledge is supposed to do. What a boring world we would live in if everything we first believed never changed. There may not be a need to seek continual knowledge, but as history is proving, this is far from true, and the thirst for knowledge must go on.

Ungraduated Call to Action

- What are some areas of lifelong learning to which you can apply yourself?
- What are some areas of old beliefs you have that may need explored?
- Is there anything in your previous learning that needs to be revisited? Why?

Chapter 5
Getting Your Mind Right

"Live as if you were to die tomorrow, learn as if you were to live forever."
~ Mahatma Gandhi ~

Wilma Rudolph was the twentieth of twenty-two children, and she was born prematurely in 1940, in Bethlehem, TN. In addition to her premature birth, she also endured many different health ailments including polio, scarlet fever, and pneumonia. As a result, her early life experiences with these challenges left her with a partially deformed left leg.

As a young child, she was encouraged by her mother. Doctors told her she would never walk again, but her mother told her she would. She had to wear leg braces to help her walk and attended physical therapy in hopes that she could one day live a normal life. Through the encouragement and support from her family, Wilma was able to take off the leg braces at the age of nine. A few years later, she was playing basketball. It's a good thing she listened more to her mother than her doctors.

Wilma went from a child whom most doctors told would not live a normal life to becoming quite a good athlete. While she was in high school, word traveled. She caught the attention of the University of Tennessee track coach, who began coaching her through her remaining high school years. She would attend college-level practices while in high school, always working to fine-tune her skill. She became so good that she never lost a high school track meet. At the age of sixteen, she tried out for and won a spot to compete in the 1956 Olympics held in Melbourne, Australia. She placed with a Bronze medal during the 4×100-meter relay.

She didn't stop with that achievement. She continued to work on her skills, enrolled at Tennessee State, and continued to win track meets at the college level. During the 1960 Olympics in Rome, she became the first woman to win three gold medals. She took first place in the 100-meter, 200-meter, and 4×100-meter relay. She was dubbed "The World's Fastest Woman," and was named the Associated Press Female of the Year.

From the little girl who would likely never walk again—to three-time Olympic Gold medalist and Female Athlete of the Year. Quite an astonishing turn of events. Was this simply a lucky break or coincidence? I think not. It had everything to do with mindset and determination. She could have believed what the experts told her, and she likely would have drifted off into a world of underachievement. But she, along with her family, framed the right mindset to persevere and redefine her future and what it was meant to be.[17]

Fixed Mindsets

Fixed mindsets are the type of thoughts that limit us and hold us back. When we live with a fixed mindset, we believe that life happens to us. We see life as uncontrollable and random. People living with a fixed mindset believe that they have little control over what's happening to them.

In this mentality, we point a finger at life and play the blame game. We tend to have a "woe is me" kind of a mentality. People in a fixed mindset often wonder if they're ever going to be able to really achieve success, happiness, and fulfillment. They see the attainment of their goals as far more difficult due to the challenges and issues that keep getting placed in front of them.

Fixed mindset beliefs look and sound like this:

- I have limited aspects in life that I am good at.
- I avoid challenges.
- Any feedback I receive on how I do something is a personal attack.
- I avoid what I don't know.
- When the going gets tough, I'd rather give in.

These types of beliefs keep us held back in life and attract more negativity to us. Have you ever known someone that is constantly talking about all the bad things in life that are happening to them? All we ever hear from these individuals is how horrible things are in their lives. There never seems to be anything good that comes to them. What most of these types of fixed-mindset people don't realize is this: their perception of their reality is perpetuating the continued outcome of the negativity. What they need is a shift in mindset.

Victims of Life's Circumstances

Fixed mindsets can really be summed up well as victim mindsets. It sounds harsh, but that is really what it boils down to. Those living within a victim mindset see themselves as victims of life's lessons and teachings. Here are some commonalities that define the victim and fixed mindset:

- Avoidance—We avoid what we don't know instead of seeking out new information or getting into new opportunities. These are avoided for the fear of the challenge or discomfort and not wanting to get outside of our comfort zones.
- Denial—We don't like feedback and often don't agree with it. We don't see ourselves as the problem but see others as the reasons for our setbacks and shortcomings.
- Resentment—When we do see success in others around us, we experience feelings of jealousy, hollowness, and the

desire for what they achieve. We make up excuses in our minds for why we can't attain the success that others have.
- Education is Finite—This is the belief that we have learned all there really is needed to exist in life. We don't feel there is enough benefit to learning more.

Growing to New Heights

Growth mindsets are the type of thinking and perspectives that empower us and bring more positivity and growth to our everyday living. In a growth mindset, we are constantly looking for feedback, learning, and embracing life's challenges. Even when the going gets tough, people in growth mindsets use those opportunities to add more experiential learning and development. There is little finger-pointing in this mindset, as the individual understands there is good that can come from life's difficult times. Growth mindsets look and sound like this:

- I can be good at most anything I put my mind to.
- I embrace challenges.
- Any feedback I receive in life can and should be used for growth and learning.
- I lean into the unknown to learn more.
- When the going gets tough, I work harder to get through and not give in.

When operating in a growth mindset, we see life as 90% within our control. The remaining 10% that happens out of our control still gives us a choice in how we respond. We look at life as happening *for* us, not happening *to* us. Romans 8:28 (NIV) says, "And we know that in all things God works for the good of those who love him, who have been called according to his purpose." The Bible teaches a growth mindset.

Many people see life as too random with too many things beyond our control. I can assure you that you can take a step back and realize that it really is your mindset that creates a lot of the negativity or positivity in your life. Here are some commonalities and behaviors that coincide with growth mindsets:

- **Be accountable.** Whatever is happening to us in life, we step back and realize that we're accountable for most things. Even in the more difficult challenges we may face, we look at how we may be bringing these issues onto our horizons.
- **Achieve.** We look at things that happen to us as really things that happen *for* us. So instead of seeing life as randomly throwing jabs and punches, we are always looking for ways to counterpunch. We see life's challenges as being here for us to grow and achieve more.
- **Embrace criticism.** We know that feedback is valuable, and we need it to improve. Everyone isn't always going to see it our way, and we don't try to please all the people we meet in life.
- **Learning is lifelong.** To stop learning is a personal choice. No matter what level of education, whether it be G. E. D. or high school diploma to an MBA or a doctorate, we know that life is always offering more opportunities from which to learn and grow.

When we operate with a growth mindset, we see the world and the many moving parts that affect us as mostly positive. When we shift our view toward this mentality, we are rewarded with more benefits, growth, and personal learnings.

The Power of Choice

The beauty of life comes down to this—we get to choose how we frame our life and the mindsets that we live with. Not only do we get to choose our mindset and belief system, but we also get to choose the food we eat, the amount of exercise we get, and how we spend the majority of our time each day. The choices we make about how to improve ourselves and how we respond to some of life's greatest adversities are at the very center of our lives whether we realize it or not. In order to make the most positive impact in our lives, we must choose to become aware. We must begin to pay attention to the choices we make.

The first step in understanding the power of choice is to take notice of the many different choices we have in a given day. Outside of any instinctive reaction, our daily decisions are all personal choices. Beginning to recognize that we are making choices every day is what gives us power. If we don't like the results we are getting in life, we have the free will to make different decisions. When we find ourselves with undesirable results, we can choose to change those outcomes.

Some of these undesirable outcomes come to us in the form of habits. Many people will try to argue that habits—both good and bad—once ingrained, are no longer choices. This simply isn't true. One of my bad habits was finding every reason to not exercise. The excuses came in abundance. Even though I hated the image in the mirror, I had gotten into the unhealthy habit of not exercising. Each day, I found a good excuse to not exercise.

Until one day I didn't.

I broke out of the routine of making excuses and feeding my rationale of not having the time. I rearranged my schedule so I could easily make forty-five minutes to an hour to exercise. I made the choices necessary to no longer feed the bad habit.

Now I have a good habit of daily exercise never missing a day. That too is a choice. I don't have to get up and exercise daily—I choose to.

Choice vs Innate Abilities

Much of my early life, I believed I was a product of circumstances. I believed that my body, genetic makeup, and mental capacity was set at a predetermined position. While I believed I could still achieve most things, I had a fixed mindset around my body and the genetics I was dealt. As we'll see in upcoming chapters, even your genetics aren't completely fixed.

There were many poor choices I made around my health and wellness, as I just assumed I would never likely be at the weight I desired or have the mental capacity needed to really excel at certain topics. I would choose to drink more and eat more because those things felt better in the moment and were justifiable by my short-term fixed mindset at the time. What resulted was years of setting myself back both mentally and physically.

I've since made great progress in both areas but often wonder how much further ahead I could be had I not made those choices based on my assumed limitations.

There are many people with good and bad innate abilities who still choose to make bad choices. They either believe that the world will cut them a break if they are having a rough time of things or that they will find their great potential because the world owes it to them. The fact of the matter is the world isn't keeping score and doesn't owe you anything based on your potential alone. The world only responds to you when you decide to take action. It responds to choices you make—in good and bad decisions, you will always get the response deserved. Maybe not overnight, but you will receive it.

When I eventually chose to move into a growth mindset, my life began taking off for the better, in so many more ways than just health and wellness. I realized that whatever abilities I was or wasn't given at birth were meaningless until I decided to make better choices that would produce the outcomes conducive to growth.

To this day, I continue to see myself as a constant work in progress, continuing to learn from every choice I make.

Choosing How to Live

Coming to the realization that you possess the power of choice is a freeing experience. When you achieve this mentality, you shift completely out of a fixed mindset and into a growth mindset. You can choose where your life will take you. You don't have to wait for the success train to come to your stop; you can be the driver of the train and take others for the ride along with you.

Challenging ourselves and stepping outside of our comfort zones can be a little scary and nerve racking. But it shows us that we are *alive*.We can step bravely into growth and discomfort or retreat into safety and complacency.

Wilma Rudolf certainly could have chosen the easy road. She could have accepted her prognosis and limited lifestyle. But instead, she chose to lean into her challenges. She decided that she wasn't going to allow life to paint her into a nice, neat corner that was labeled "disadvantaged and unfortunate." She persisted and persevered through all the odds and wrote her own chapters in life on her own terms. It is far easier to stay in a fixed zone of comforts than to step outside into the world of growth and opportunity. Which life will you choose for yourself?

Ungraduated Call to Action

- What are some areas of your life in which you are living within a fixed mindset?
- How can you shift these limiting beliefs into more of a growth mindset?
- Make one commitment that you are going to begin to do every day from this day forward that is going to benefit you in your goals. Share it with an accountability partner.

Chapter 6

Generating Personal Abundance & Happiness

"It is the preoccupation with possessions, more than anything else, that prevents us from living freely and nobly."
~ Bertrand Russell ~

The year was 1848. A gentleman by the name of James Marshall had been working to build a sawmill by the current-day city of Sacramento, CA. Suddenly, he saw something that appeared to be metal, glowing a yellowish radiant tint in the earth where he had been digging. Marshall had struck upon gold. Even in a time well ahead of advanced communication technology, it didn't take long for the rumors to spread. Within a few weeks, tens of thousands of people seeking to strike it rich flocked to the area.

People became so enamored with the possibility of living a life of riches, they abandoned their ships, businesses, homes, and even their families in hopes of finding the precious metal that humankind deems so valuable. San Francisco ballooned from a village of eighty buildings to a city with tens of thousands of buildings. Entire towns were left abandoned for the hopes and dreams of finding life-changing wealth.

Over the next few years, what resulted was more than 300,000 gold seekers who became known as "the 49ers" as they all sought to punch their "get rich quick" ticket to their own Super Bowl of life! There is your history lesson on the National Football League team named the San Francisco 49ers—just in case you weren't already aware. But I digress. What these 49ers of the 1800s were seeking was what they believed would change their lives and make them happy.

What is often not discussed with the Gold Rush was the ramifications it had on the local Native American population. So great was the desire to get rich, there was no regard for the existing population. Native Americans saw their land and rivers polluted by the miners, they contracted diseases from the large influx of so many foreign people, and they lost their grounds for hunting and farming. Some were even taken as slaves while their women were carried away to be sold. Those who tried to protect their lands were killed off, leaving the remaining to starve or die of new diseases. All in the name of a yellow metal deemed to have value.

Some tribes were so perplexed by the desire to obtain the precious metal that they began to pray over chests of gold. Their belief was that the invaders must have seen the precious metal as some sort of god. Why would anyone go to such lengths to acquire it?

Living in a Material World

Who else while reading that subheading can literally hear Madonna's voice in their head? Ha ha! Me, too.

But, in all seriousness, we live in a material world. We are marketed to incessantly over and over throughout our day. Each company seeks to exchange a good for a share of our gold. It is easy to get caught up in the confusion of what we need to drive true happiness and prosperity. Much of our lives, we are told we need to grow up, finish school, buy a car, then buy a house, furnish that house, have children, provide for our children, and onward the cycle goes.

We define ourselves by our material possessions, and they often define us. We have already learned through the Ungraduation process that we are not our labels, but trying to wrap our minds around what drives happiness can be a daunting task.

People often hear that money and other material things don't generate happiness, but do we really believe this? Yes, it is true, we all need some basic essentials, and we do need money in order to secure them. But there is so much more to life than simply acquiring more stuff. The things we want to purchase may bring us short-term joy, but we don't gain long-lasting happiness from them. We all need to take care of our basic needs: food, water, shelter, and good health. After all, we can't be of any service to others if we don't first take care of ourselves.

Let's define exactly what material things are:

- Material things are possessions we purchase or acquire in this physical world.
- Material things consist of houses, cars, clothes, jewelry, technology, books, boats, or just about any other "physical thing" you could imagine yourself wanting.
- Material things are anything you can envision yourself spending money on.

We need some of the abovementioned material things. We need a reliable car to get us to and from work or from point A to point B so that we can earn a paycheck and get food and other necessities. This paradigm is beginning to change with more people working from home and ordering online, but for the vast majority of us, having a reliable car is still an absolute necessity. We all need to be able to put food on our tables and clothes on our backs. It is expected to have a safe home with items of comfort for your lifestyle.

Where the misalignment begins is when we begin to center our happiness around the need to acquire more things beyond our basic needs. Don't get me wrong; the occasional reward for a job well done is not bad, but it shouldn't be the main method of motivation. This is how we form addictions to acquiring more things. Many of us work hard and do deserve a reward from time to time, so don't misunderstand me. I do feel life and some of the materialistic aspects of it are meant to be experienced, but it just needs put into proper perspective.

We can tend to quickly fall out of alignment when we begin to think that getting a greater number of material things in our lives is the primary goal. As a society, we are quick to rank ourselves against others by what type of car we have and whether or not we have the newest televisions or smart devices. This is where the trap of keeping up with the Joneses comes into play. We quickly are made to believe that in order to be happy, we need to compete with others and ensure that we have what they have. Otherwise, if we don't have the latest and greatest, then we must be failing in some way.

As I type this chapter, I'm still rocking with my iPhone 7. Even though I'm five or six versions behind the latest model, my current phone does everything I need it to. It has enough storage for all my apps and programs, and it is still able to take all the latest iOS updates. I realize one day I'll need to purchase a new phone, but why spend the money each year on a new device that is not vastly superior to the one I currently have?

I give a lot of credit to my wife for how she helped instill some of these perspectives in me early on in our relationship. I was far from perfect, having been brought up in life with very little. Each time I would fall into some money, I was tempted to splurge on toys and the latest gadgets. She was great about teaching me the lesson no one else would: if you don't have the money to pay for it now, then you don't buy it. Those darn credit card companies. As Charles Dickens wrote, "It was the best of times, it was the worst of times...." That about summed up my early learnings around credit.

Here is a thought I'll leave you with before we move on to discussing ways to get out of a materialistic mindset and move toward a happiness mindset. Imagine your dream car. Picture it in your head. The year, make, model, and color. Then imagine you are given the complete amount of money it would cost to purchase the car, but it came with one caveat. Each time you took it out for a spin, you could only do so when no one was watching. Would you still buy it? Would you retain the desire to have it? This perspective might help reframe whether you are purchasing something because you need it and it makes you happy, or you're buying it for the satisfaction of ego and the need to impress others. It helps to understand your wants and desires in this manner before you make those impulsive purchases—large and small.

Needy Humans

Before we can shift into gear around how we can drive more systemic happiness in our lives, we must understand there are some requirements we must have in place first. I'm not sure when I was first introduced to Maslow's Heirarchy of Needs, but when I was, I remember I was likely in the third rung, love and belonging. I had the first few levels locked down with physiological needs and safety needs. What I wanted and sought was social connection and appreciation.

Without trying to give too much of a psychological dissertation here, Maslow's Hierarchy of Needs really spells out the human story and perspective quite well.

In order to achieve higher levels of happiness in life, we need to fill base-level needs first. As humans, we can't level up toward more fulfillment in life if we don't first satisfy the lower levels. While

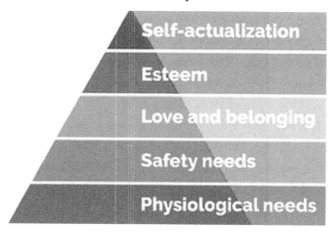

Maslow's Heiarchy of Needs has been debated, and some argue against his paradigm, I believe there to be more evidence for it versus against it as I look at life through my own experiences.

At the base level, we have physiological needs. This level includes the needs for food, shelter, water, sleep, and clothing. Failure to attain those items often leads to the inability to even focus on reproduction and the continuation of our species. Once we have those basic needs met, we can move up to safety needs. Upon reaching this level, we satisfy our personal security, income, necessary living resources, health, and property. It isn't until we can guarantee those first two levels of needs that we can begin to think about connection and the love and belonging aspect of our needs. Here we begin to look for social relationships and seek acceptance with friends, family, and other intimate relationships. Most of the developed world find themselves at this level. Sadly, however, even in developed countries, there are still too many that can't achieve this level for various reasons.

> Little do the power hungry realize, the truly powerful in this world know through love they conquer all.

Once we move into the esteem level of Maslow's Hierarchy of Needs, we begin to feel more free. At this point, we begin to really drive our lives around attaining more happiness, excitement, and zest from life. This is where much of humanity gets stuck. We often don't see the trap that exists in front of us, that attaining more stuff isn't going to make us happy. We may achieve some short-term recognition from friends, family, and peers, but quickly the excitement fades, and we're on to the need for the next *fix* and trying to find that all-important status in life.

It is when we can look inward deeply enough to realize that we have the money, status, recognition, and success we need in life that we can begin to wonder how we can leave more of a lasting impact for others rather than just for ourselves. At this point, it begins to be more about how we drive real happiness through self-worth than material gains.

Don't Worry—Be Happy Now!

Now with a renewed perspective on our human needs, we can look at what it will take to Ungraduate from living in a world driven by material wants and desires to a world that is more fueled through our own self-actualization and empowerment. We can decide our happiness and won't need to attain it through the material world.

The first bucket of life we will look to Ungraduate from is how we visually consume throughout the day. Everywhere we look, our eyes feed signals to our brains. What we are viewing and where we are putting our attention determine what messages our brains receive.

Visual Inputs

Begin by limiting television. Let me just break that word down a little bit closer for you Tell-a-Vision. Did you ever think of TV in that manner? Makes you wonder what marketing genius came up with the name. They were spot-on with that one. The TV is constantly *telling us a vision* of what the marketers want us to think and feel. Let's take it one step further. What are the things on TV called? That's right—say it with me now . . . *programs*! Wait a second. So we're watching *programs* on a device that is meant to *tell-a-vision*? I don't know about you, but I don't take kindly to being programmed by other people's visions. I like to march to the beat of my own drum. So just beginning with limiting TV is one great way to get to break free of materialistic traps.

I'm not saying all TV is bad. There are great documentaries and other aspects of good in television. But a large portion of it is aimed to ensnare us into other people's visions and marketing gimmicks. If you don't watch as often, you won't fall for the trap! If there is that one show you just love to immerse yourself in, then see if you can just record it. That way, you can still get your fix but fast forward through the marketing.

In addition to cutting back on television, reduce your intake of broadcast news. Not only will your mood be better, but you'll avoid the advertisements that center around feeding the networks that have the higher-rated shows. What really drives the marketing agencies at the news networks are their prime time shows that get the most airtime. If there are any honest networks out there, they would tell you that what really matters most to them is marketing dollars. That is where they earn their paycheck, and those paychecks come to them from viewers like you who are tuned in to your favorite talking head on the nightly news.

How about reading? Well, that all depends on where you're doing your reading. If at all possible, try to limit reading on your laptop or smart devices. There is too much temptation to browse sites while online, and what do you usually see on most websites? That's right, more advertising aimed at snatching a share of your hard-earned cash. Plus, we fall victim to mindless internet wandering that sometimes leads to mindless purchasing. Shopping from our pajamas is just too easy to do. So limit your reading to hardcopy books or e-readers. Even magazines are loaded with advertising aimed to get you wanting that new car or latest tech gadget that they ever so eloquently try to get you to believe you cannot do without—or you'll be unhappy! Books don't come with advertising, at least not the type that you're going to get in your face on every turn of a page or after every ten minutes like commercials do on TV.

Monitoring Your Urges

Avoid big-box retailers and malls as much as possible. Frequenting these places is just another way that we trip ourselves up to thinking we want or need more things. These places rarely only have just what we need. They love to advertise the new shiny objects that they want us to indulge in.

Obviously, we will need to shop, but what I'm referring to is when we are looking to blow off steam or take some time off. Find a better place to go for a walk, such as a park, beach, trails through the woods, or around your neighborhood. Reconnecting with anything outdoors is a far better way to put your mind at ease than the sensory overload of more items flashing in front of you.

It also helps to keep track of all the different times you feel the urge to make purchases. Whether that is when you are browsing the internet or doing any in-person shopping, notice it. One best practice is to open up a phone app for taking notes and quickly note the day and time along with what you are thinking of purchasing. By tracking the times we feel urges to make purchases, we can become more aware. By becoming more aware, we begin to take back control of our mind and recenter ourselves around driving actual happiness, not short-term fixes.

When you do find yourself needing to make a purchase, see if it is something that you can buy used. My wife is an expert at this. Not only does she find amazing deals all the time, but she is also constantly complimented on it. From clothes to antique tables and chairs that she has refurbished, she is continually making the old and unwanted into the new and desirable. Not only does it save money, but it can also be a fulfilling hobby that generates self-worth and happiness.

Organizing & Tracking

Another way to Ungraduate from habitual spending on items is to make lists. The first type of list is centered around items you really believe you need or want. If you can't seem to get past the desire to purchase something, put it on your monthly purchase list. This can again be done relatively easily on a smart device, or we simply could go with old-school scraps of paper or index cards. Either way, having a place where we can look back over a thirty-day period is the goal here.

What we aim to accomplish is generating a list of items we believe we need. At the end of the month, if you genuinely feel you still need the item and have the funds to do it, then make the purchase. However, in many cases, you'll find you were suffering a short-term impulse. You will see that after the desire to want to purchase the item passes, you really didn't need to make that purchase. This aims to keep your buying on impulse down and trains your mind to realize what you genuinely need in life, and what is likely not necessary.

Next is the aspect of gratitude lists. This is something I cannot emphasize the value of enough. I was never a big journal guy, but as I've learned to make gratitude lists, I'm finding so much more happiness. Whether you choose this routine to begin your day or end your day, make three bullet points for what you are grateful for. They can be things that you're looking forward to in your day or things you were thankful to experience. They can sometimes be the same things over and over, but most often you'll find many different things that come in and out of your life generate a lot of gratitude. Just the overall positive approach of daily gratitude is enough to cause mindset shifts in the field of energy that we all live and operate within to bring happiness and positivity into our lives over the negative.

The next step centers around organization. If you aren't a very organized person to begin with, making some time to declutter your living space will go a long way to generate more happiness. Not only has a lot of stuff lying around been proven to cause higher levels of stress and anxiety, it also feels better to be in a cleaner, more organized living space. This goes for your personal vehicle, too. Invest some time to clean out closets on a biannual basis, organize your home office monthly, and ensure your living quarters haven't become too disorganized with stuff. If you can, part ways with some of the extra stuff that you have collected over the years. Not only can you sometimes make someone else's life better by donating, but you can also make a few extra bucks by having a garage sale.

What selling, donating, or getting rid of the extra stuff in your life does is it shows you just how infrequently we really use the things we have at home. It will help you more into the future to think twice before buying more stuff as you see how frequently you are throwing away, donating, or selling your items at home.

Blazing a True Path to More Happiness

Now that we have defined and called out some of the key points concerning material possessions, we can reframe how to generate more abundance, personal satisfaction, and happiness. Once we can recognize the possible pitfalls, it all comes down to what a lot of other aspects of our lives come down to—choice. This can't be overstated. Every day of our lives, we make thousands of choices. Researchers at Cornell University estimate that human beings on average make around 35,000 remotely conscious choices a day.[18] Each decision carries its own set of positive or negative outcomes. Here are some key decisions that can really help put us into a better state of overall abundance and happiness:

> Always remember no matter how bleak a circumstance may look, no one can take away the power of choice and meaning we have within ourselves.

Choose to think positively. Not everyone is wired this way, but I promise if you work on it, you're going to attract more positivity into your world. Your view of life and the world around you matters. How you frame it determines how you experience it. (Principle of Mentalism)

Bring small pleasures into your day. Become mindful of what you enjoy doing, and find a way to work those small things into your everyday activities. For example, if you enjoy being outside, take the laptop outside for some time during the workday. Find ways to integrate into your daily routine small activities you enjoy. You'll find yourself doing more of what you enjoy each day over what you don't. (Principle of Rhythm)

Practice kindness. Simply being kind and generous will go further for most than they realize. You don't need to walk around buying everyone their morning coffee, but find ways to generate random acts of kindness without the expectation of reciprocation. You'll find happiness in simply doing this, and you'll find the Universe continually gives back to you tenfold. (Principle of Cause & Effect)

Show more love. This is something that we typically reserve only for our close relatives, and sadly in some cases not nearly enough. When we express more love outwardly, we're going to find less room for feelings of fear, regret, and despair. Who doesn't need a little more love in their life? Balance your right brain (emotion) to your (left brain) practical self, and don't be afraid to show love. If you want more love, give more love. (Principle of Gender)

Eat healthfully & exercise routinely. We've all heard of the endorphins we release when we exercise. There is so much good that comes from eating healthfully and building an exercise routine. It's hard to feel love for others when we don't love ourselves. Our bodies are connected to our minds. We can literally think ourselves sick or healthy. More on this later, but for now, realize the importance of investing in your body and health. (Principle of Rhythm)

Get in flow state. As you work through your day, eliminate as many distractions as possible. When you are working on a project, enable the Do Not Disturb setting on your phone and laptop. Block time on your calendar. You will feel deeper satisfaction in a job well done by being able to use your flow state to its fullest while you are at your highest levels of attention. We constantly are in flux with energy with the highs and lows of our productivity throughout the day. Be aware of this. (Principle of Polarity)

Know yourself. As you work to become more mindful of things that make you happy and begin to choose more activities and functions you enjoy, you will learn more about where to spend your time and with whom. This is where you begin to make more time for the people around you that *you jive with*, and those that you don't, you begin to eliminate or make less time for. The more you're aware of yourself, the more you'll attract similar people to you—happy and abundant people. (Principle of Vibration)

You now have your ticket to your gold treasure chest. Your real treasure, that is—the ability you have to understand how framing up your mind matters in your happiness. We have more abilities than we sometimes realize to manifest our own abundance and happiness. The best part of it all is we don't need to wait for the next gold rush for riches; it all exists right in front of us. We just have to choose to see it.

Ungraduated Call to Action

- Where have you given too much time and attention to "material things" in your life?
- What are some aspects of your life that you could never do without? What and why?
- What are some of the biggest mindset shifts you need to make to bring more happiness and abundance into your life?

Part 3
The Connection of Body & Mind

Chapter 7
Self-Synchronization

"We are not human beings having a spiritual experience. We are spiritual beings having a human experience."
~ Pierre Teilhard de Chardin ~

By all accounts from the outside looking in, Robert Monroe was an overall average human being. He aimed to make a living for himself and his family like many other Americans in the post-World-War-II era. However, in his midforties, he would begin to experience phenomena in his life that were anything but average. Robert would find himself in the middle of the night out of his body. Come again? Yes, that is right—he would see himself lying in bed and consciously and freely experiencing life from an altered state of consciousness. By all accounts, he was not *in his body*.

Even though this may sound like an episode straight out of *The Twilight Zone*, it is all very true and well documented. Beginning around 1958, Robert began to document his experiences. You can likely imagine how it had to feel to "wake up" and see your body lying in bed below. His first thought was, *My God—I'm dead!* but he was far from the Spirit in the sky that night, as he would awake and snap back into his body as if nothing irregular had occurred. These events continued and created fear and confusion, as he wanted and needed answers for this strange abnormality he had developed.

Fearful that he had a brain tumor or some other terminal illness, he had his doctor give him every test in the book to determine what, if anything, could be going on. He was far too afraid to talk to most people about his experiences for fear of being locked away in an insane asylum. But test after test continued to prove that he was healthy for his age.

His doctor would remind him that he likely needed to cut back on the smoking and he could certainly afford to trim an inch or so off his waistline, but that wasn't too different from the average Joe.

Discouraged by not having a satisfactory level of reasoning or explanation, he became resigned to make the most of his situation and generate as much self-discovery and learning about his unfortunate and terrifying almost-nightly occurrences.

These occurrences began to happen with some regularity. He began to write down his experiences and even noted when they would occur, to prove that he wasn't dreaming. For example, he and some friends decided that they would test his theory that he was actually able to exit his body and still "move about" consciously. Upon a successful event, he would describe occurrences with those acquaintances. During one of his test episodes, he exited his body and describes it in the following passage:

> The first thing I saw was a boy walking along and tossing a baseball in the air and catching it. A quick shift, and I saw a man trying to put something in the back seat of a car, a large sedan. The thing was an awkward looking device that I interpreted to be a small car with wheels and electric motor. The man twisted and turned the device and finally got it into the back seat of the car and slammed the door. Another quick shift, and I was standing by a table. There were people sitting at the table, and dishes covered it. One person was dealing what looked like large white playing cards around to the others at the table. I thought it strange to play cards at a table so covered in dishes and wondered about the overall size and whiteness of the cards. Another quick shift, and I was over the city streets, about five hundred

feet high, looking for "home." Then I spotted the radio tower, and remembered the motel was close to the tower, and almost instantly, I was back in my body.

Here is the importance in this story from Robert Monroe's book—he had an intuitive feeling that his morning experience had something to do with a few of his close friends. Their names were Mr. and Mrs. Agnew Bahnson. He went to visit them the same evening and asked them about his event and what he saw while out of body. He asked them about their son and what he may have been doing that morning between 8:00 AM and 8:30 AM. Mr. Bahnson responded that he was going to school and walking there while tossing and catching his baseball. Next, Robert asked Mr. Bahnson about what he was loading into his car. Astounded, Mr. Bahnson replied that he was trying to load a Van Degraff generator into his car. That was the awkward device Robert described as looking like a "small car with wheels and an electric motor."

Next, Mr. Monroe asked Mrs. Bahnson about the table and large white playing cards. She went on to explain that they had awoken late that morning and she had decided to bring the mail to the table at breakfast and pass out their letters to the members of her family.

Robert Monroe went on to describe many other scenes like this in which he documented factual supporting evidence in his first book, *Journeys Out of the Body*. To him, this was significant verifiable evidence that was what he was experiencing was real. There are numerous other amazing stories of validation of Robert's experiences that you can read for yourself in his three books on the topic of out-of-body experiences or OBEs.

From even before Robert Monroe's revelations, and certainly after, there have been many studies conducted by different research agencies ranging from the CIA to Robert's own formation of the Monroe Institute, which specializes in altered states of consciousness and different forms of remote viewing and OBEs.

The Conscious Mind Connection

Once we begin to realize that at our essence, we are energy—spirit, encapsulated by flesh—we can begin to tune our minds for greater life purposes. Our spirt is connected to and a part of an energy consciousness, and we can begin the work of balancing the trinity of mind, spirit, and body. All things begin in the mind with thought. Through focus and motivation to action, we can focus our energy to drive our consciousness into action. This happens at a physical and nonphysical level (with or without a body). How motivated we are to manifest our thought into action dictates the outcome we experience within our physical realities.

> If we can get ourselves into proper mind, body, and spirit alignment, then we can begin moving up the ladder of consciousness on our way to becoming our best selves possible.

The trinity of mind, spirit, and body can also be conceptualized as thought, emotion, and action. Many of the problems we generate for ourselves begin in our own thoughts. The same can be said for our victories and positive outcomes. Whether we realize it or not, we are constantly downloading into our physical beings either positive or negative thoughts. If we want to fix a problem, we must fix the thinking first. It is a very empowering position to be in once we discover we are not victims of circumstances—rather, we are creating them.

When we begin to understand that the brain is a powerful transmitter that is connected to the consciousness, all life and knowledge the Universe has to offer us can become available. For much of modern history, scientists have labeled the brain as the number-one communicator for the body. We have been taught that the neurons in our brain are connected to all the nerves and muscles within our bodies. It is through these electronic pathways to the brain that our bodies respond to thought and action. A lot of this action occurs without any thinking at all—fortunately—such as breathing, digestion, and other necessities of human functioning. The brain is certainly one of the most important organs in our body, and few would attempt to dispute that fact. However, new scientific studies are beginning to shed light on another major organ that we all realize the importance of but are beginning to discover new learnings on its connection to the brain: the heart.

The Heart Connection

Besides the obvious importance of the function the heart serves, there are other importances that are beginning to weave their way into the fabric of the mind–body connection. New scientific discoveries are showing that besides the important function of pumping blood through the body, the heart is very much like a brain itself.

At the start of life, the heart beats before the brain is formed. When the brain dies, the heart will still beat so long as it has oxygen. The heart has 40,000 sensory neurites and the ability to process, learn, and remember just like the brain, essentially giving it the ability to act independently from the brain. The heart sends meaningful messages of its own throughout our bodies. It has also been discovered that the heart has its own level of emotions. Through the field of neurocardiology, science is discovering more about the intuitive nature of the heart. We can maximize this understanding for our betterment and that of those around us.

The Heartmath Institute has become a leading research institution studying heart–brain synchronization. According to Research Director Dr. Rollin McCraty, "Coherence is the state when the heart, mind, and emotions are in energetic alignment and cooperation. It is a state that builds resilience." What exactly is this coherence, or synchronization, as we'll refer to it? It is the ability for the feeling and emotions within the heart to send signals to the brain, which then of course the brain relays to the body. When we find ourselves in levels of lower conscious thought such as fear, anger, or jealousy—our hearts send erratic or incoherent signals back to the brain. When we find ourselves in emotions such as love, gratitude, and appreciation—our hearts send signals that are in coherence within these higher levels of consciousness, and our brains then send those signals through our bodies.

When we can send more higher-level consciousness signals from our hearts to our brains, we find ourselves within a state that is referred to as physiological synchronization. When we can build up these higher-level consciousness signals from our hearts to our brains, our bodies respond in different levels of brain wave activity to support lowered blood pressure, stress relief, and other positive outcomes for ourselves.[19]

A Personal State of Panic

Unfortunately, like many people, I have had firsthand experience with anxiety and panic attacks. In my twenties, I suffered from high blood pressure and high levels of anxiety. So bad, actually, that they resulted in trips to doctors and hospitals, as I wasn't sure if I was having anxiety attacks or heart attacks.

One evening while living at our home in Florida, I jumped up from the couch and insisted my wife put her hand on my chest. With all my might, I tried to calm the panic in my voice as I asked her why my heart would be palpitating and racing for no apparent reason. I paced back and forth, taking deep breaths and trying to get my mind right—telling myself, "This can't be happening. I'm too young to be having a heart attack—but what if I am?" Sweat beaded on my forehead as I felt a wet and clammy sensation all over my body. I tried to decide what to do. My wife asked if I wanted to go to the hospital.

Stubborn and confused, I attempted with all my mental might to stop whatever it was. I didn't feel any pain, but to have my heart racing as if I had just completed a footrace while I was only siting on the couch simply made no sense to me. Slowly, the pulsation of the blood rushing to my head began to calm, and my body seemed to begin returning to a state of normality. The sweating stopped, and I felt as if I had quelled the strange attack of anxiety against me.

These episodes would happen a few times a month, sometimes more, resulting in a visit to have an echocardiogram and electrocardiogram (EKG). I remember my body tensing up and heart rate increasing as the tests were performed. That was a common occurrence in my young adult life. Visits to doctors' offices or hospitals always put me on edge. Often in these visits, the nurses had to take second readings of my blood pressure because of how high it would read as I simply sat in the office. It was as if I was in a constant state of panic and fear—I did not know why, but I could very much feel it.

The nurse taking the readings of the tests gave me her findings as I was hooked up to the machine that gave the readouts. "Nothing wrong with your heart—perfectly normal rhythm and beating," as she pointed to the heartbeat that was being produced by the muscle beating away in my chest. As relieved as I was to hear that, I had been so sure something had to be wrong. The bouts of elevated heart rate for no reason, feelings of not being able to breathe as if my chest were being weighed down with cinder blocks, and feeling of mental blanking out that would occur during the anxiety attacks made me feel hopeless. I had been sure that something was wrong with my heart, and even receiving good news that it was healthy, I was left with more questions than answers.

Heart & Brain Synchronization

As I grew into my early thirties and discovered meditation, slowly and over time, I could feel myself beginning to have a different presence or awareness. I had always heard that meditation was good for you—but really didn't know why or understand its positive effects.

There are many different forms of meditation. I read a few books on mediation and enjoyed the type in which you consciously scan your body and aim to feel deeply into different sections of the body. I would often focus on my heart and feel for the pulses as they would pump blood through my body. The feeling I received from twenty minutes was so calming and euphoric.

While I didn't meditate every day, slowly and over time, the anxiety attacks ceased. My blood pressure checks became normal, and it has been nearly fifteen years since I last experienced an anxiety attack. My doctor visits show normal to very good blood pressure every time I visit. Through a conscious connection from my heart to my brain, I have corrected issues that many receive medication for. I am not saying that all medication is bad or unnecessary, but I am forever grateful that I have been able to solve this personal issue without the need for any antianxiety drugs or other medicines.

I'm assuming you'd like to know how to conduct this heart-to-brain synchronization. Great news—it's very simple. First, get into a comfortable position sitting or lying down. Next, slow your breathing—take slow deep breaths in and slow deep breaths out for about a minute or so. Then, begin to focus your attention on your heart. Feel the heart beating while you're thinking the following thoughts: *Love, Compassion, Gratitude,* and *Care*. Do this for five minutes or longer. You can do this each day at any time of the day that best suits you.

The only caveat to this is you must genuinely feel thoughts of love, care, compassion, and gratitude. Think of all the things you have in your life that you are grateful for. We all have these things but rarely put in the time on a daily basis to reflect on them. Express real mental love and care for the world and those around you—despite our many differences.

Then express real compassion for the countless situations that should demand our compassion. You can personalize this to your own life or keep it high level with that of the world. The thoughts you generate matter not, only that you are sincere in thinking them.

This simple daily act will get you on your way to a very important step in the ability to connect physically and electromagnetically from your heart to your brain. The benefits go well beyond physical health, calmness, and lowered anxiety, as we will soon discover.

My Own Personal Out-of-Body Experience

I was in my midtwenties. I awoke one morning like I never had before in my life. I was frozen motionless. Quickly, fear and panic set in. Was I paralyzed? Had I somehow broken my neck while sleeping? I could see all around me, but the only things I could move were my eyes. I was not able to speak or move any muscle whatsoever.

Suddenly, I began to experience what felt like some sort of presence creeping over me. It felt heavy, as if it was bearing down on me. More fear and panic began to set in, and I may have been able to muster a couple whimpers, even though in my mind, I was screaming at the top of my lungs. I was begging for my wife to notice and shake me from the horrific moment, but I was doomed to continue to sink into my own bed, completely overtaken and pushing away whatever was trying to take over my body. In that moment, the only thing I could think of to do was to say a prayer. The only prayer I had been taught to memorize was The Lord's Prayer.

Suddenly and miraculously, I began to gain back a sensation of movement in my body, and slowly, I began to feel as if whatever presence had been around me was gone. With a few more moments, I had complete control back of my body, and the horrifying ordeal was over.

I now know this was an experience of sleep paralysis, but it had never happened to me before and has not happened since. It was this one instance only, and it sent me on quite the journey of self-exploration and a need for discovering why and how this happened to me. At the time, I was quite convinced that a demon of some sort was trying to torment me or possess me.

Studying Out-of-Body Experiences

That one experience led me down so many rabbit trails of discovery. I learned about and studied out-of-body experiences, near death experiences, clairvoyance, consciousness, and remote viewing.

There are different theories that exist explaining that our consciousness (soul) leaves our body each night when we sleep. The belief is that our consciousness stays tethered to our physical reality until we no longer are alive within this physical experience.

Many believe our consciousness leaves our body each night, and that is what is responsible for the generation of many of our dreams. Upon waking, that consciousness is then brought back from the nonphysical realms into the physical reality we all experience upon waking each day.

The night of my sleep paralysis, was it possible that somehow my brain had awakened before my consciousness had returned? I know it sounds wildly unimaginable, but these types of experiences happen more often than many may think.

That personal experience was the catalyst I needed to begin a very deep and long mission of self-discovery I continue to this day. Through meditation and attempting out-of-body experiences, even more personal truths have been brought before me. I certainly still have questions, but I no longer simply put blind faith in anything. Life has given me the experiences I needed in order to answer questions, yet also ironically keep myself growing and yearning for more answers.

Almost There

Another personal experience that was breathtaking and awe-inspiring for me happened after a few months of practicing and attempting out-of-body experiences. I woke in the middle of the night to a complete vibration pulsating up and down my body. It was like nothing I had ever experienced before. It was as if my entire body had been encapsulated inside of a large church bell and was pulsating with every ring. I could feel the energy moving up and down my spine almost like I was a large conductor for electricity. I heard a loud roaring in my ears.

I began focusing my attention away from my body, and slowly I began to feel lighter. Everything in my field of vision appeared black and white. I don't know if that was due to it being 3 AM in a dark room, or if it was simply the visionary input received as the consciousness leaves the body. Regardless, as I began feeling higher, I decided I wanted to see if I could "roll over" and see myself in bed. What I saw next I will never forget.

There in bed I saw my body and the bodies of my wife and our three little chihuahuas. My wife and the three dogs had what I only can describe as a white aura outline around them while my body was dark without any outline. Could this have been representative of my consciousness (soul) having left my body while viewing others with their energy consciousness still tethered within their bodies?

I couldn't contain my excitement and quickly found myself jumping back up in bed. My wife, somewhat startled, asked me if I was OK. I only responded with, "Did you feel any vibrating?"

Half asleep, she replied, "No. What are you talking about?"

With that, I excitedly told her we'd discuss in the morning what I had just experienced.

For most people, that would be a completely terrifying experience. Thankfully, I had read of it in my studies, knowing that it is often an experience one has before their consciousness exits their body. The difference being, I was awake and conscious.

Most people drift away to sleep and awake without noticing anything. The body has a way of ensuring this process happens unnoticed before we drift off to sleep, but with effort and practice, we can prompt our consciousness to stay aware while the body begins to fall asleep. This is the jumping-off point where conscious out-of-body experiences begin. There are far more reports, readings, and inquiries today than existed in Robert Monroe's day.

Slowly, humankind is inching toward more understanding of consciousness and what exactly happens to it when we awake and go to sleep. I have had my own experiences; perhaps you may have had them as well and are just unsure of what they are. Most people push aside these instances as weird dreams and forget about them. I can promise you, when someone does have one of these experiences, you can very clearly tell what a dream is, and what is not. Believe me when I tell you, my experiences were not dreams.

Search for Higher Meaning

I realize these stories and experiences generate a lot of questions. I can only tell my story, and I'm sure many people have different versions of their own strange experiences in life. My story is a part of my own Ungraduation and personal journey of truth. My experiences were just a part of a set of great achievements in my journey of self-discovery as life put the evidence right in front of me to some of the questions I had been asking. Without a doubt, I know that we are far more than our just our physical bodies. Personally, I needed these experiences to generate my own truth.

What I have learned in my own personal discovery and through the help of my wife is that religion and our relationship with whatever higher power we believe in is a very personal matter. Each of us is meant to experience the Source, Universe, God, our Higher Selves, in the way that makes sense for us.

I wouldn't change the way I have found my own truths—I am sure it was the path I was meant to walk in order to learn and experience the many different perspectives that have led me to my own personal awakening. What we may very well simply need more of is for the potential of all of humankind to seek out their own personal perspectives of life and the reason behind the meaning of life. We don't need to fit ourselves into any particular belief system.

We can and should write our own beliefs—our own personal system of faith through which we explore. Each of us is on a very special path of personal awakening that we will experience when ready. Fighting to learn and understand your faith is a part of your Ungraduation into higher levels of thinking and self-empowerment. That is the beauty of it It's up to you to decide.

Whether it is through having spontaneous OBEs like Robert Monroe had to endure to figure out his own truths of life and existence, or if it's just through good ol' fashioned faith and belief—you get to decide what you believe. I encourage you to continue to Ungraduate from the beliefs that may have been forced upon you and formulate your own based on your own truth and life experiences. The one thing I think we can all agree on is that we're all going to be "out of body" one day.

Ungraduated Call to Action

- Where do you want to understand more about human consciousness and the soul? What questions exist that merit deeper exploration?
- Take these questions and meditate on them for ten minutes a day—put out the intentions of "needing" to find these answers—then pay attention to what life puts in front of you.
- Practice the "Mind / Heart" meditation one time daily before getting out of bed or before going to sleep each night. Record how you feel after three weeks of this practice.

Chapter 8

Thinking Yourself Healthy

"There are no constraints on the human mind, no walls around the human spirit, no barriers to our progress except those we ourselves erect."
~ Ronald Reagan ~

It's often hard to be happy in life if we aren't at our best health. Have you ever heard of thinking yourself sick or thinking yourself well? We often hear how powerful the mind is, but I'm not quite sure how many people truly understand its power. We've already established there is energy in thought. Now we will discuss that thought connection within your body and the ability for mind–body healing.

Effects of Placebos and Nocebos

Most of us have heard of the placebo effect. It's when patients are not told they are getting something as simple as a sugar pill, and they often have miraculous recovery in their ailments as if they have been given the actual drug. This is due to patients thinking they will receive a positive benefit but being unaware they haven't been given the real drug. But have you ever heard of the nocebo effect? The nocebo effect is when patients are given a prescription or pill that they believe produces a negative outcome, when in fact they are given nothing more than a water or salt pill—and still the expected outcome occurs. *Placebo* and *nocebo* come from the Latin, *placebo* meaning "I will please" and *nocebo* meaning "I will harm."

There have been numerous studies that demonstrate the placebo and nocebo effects. In one controlled study, patients were told they would be participating in a new chemotherapy study. In the study, the control patients were given saline as their nocebo. Of them, 30% had their hair fall out from nothing more than salt water, simply because their mind knew the supposed outcome. In another study, volunteers were told they would experience a mild electric shock that would pass through their heads and may cause a headache. Despite no electric current ever being passed through their heads, two thirds of them reported developing a headache.

The same experiment can work as both a placebo and a nocebo. Take for example a test involving candidates that believed they had allergic reactions to certain foods. They were given an injection and told that it contained these allergens, even though it did not. The injection was actually saline, but it generated reactions in many of the candidates. The examiners then gave the test candidates another injection of saline, telling them it would neutralize the allergic reaction, and in many cases, it did just that.[20]

A lot of the situations involving placebos and nocebos involve pills or injections, yet there are some that even involve interpretation from those in authority, and sometimes by accident. One such case was recorded in a cardiac ward at a large Catholic hospital in the United States, in which a cardiologist observed that one of his patients had taken a turn for the worse and was likely soon to die.

A priest was called to administer last rites but by mistake went to the patient next to the dying man. With an impressive level of authority, he read the last rites to the wrong man, who promptly died within fifteen minutes.

The other man, who was dying, survived for another four days.[21]

These are just a smattering of the many examples that show that our minds are producing effects in our bodies that we often don't even realize. It exemplifies the fact that what we think really does affect our bodies and our health. Our brain's ability to formulate our realities is real—so real that it helps us determine our health. This fact merits our attention and further understanding so that we can learn to keep healthy thoughts that will keep illness and other unhealthy symptoms out of our lives.

Needing a New Pair of "Genes"

We were once taught that we were stuck with the genes we were born with. High blood pressure and high cholesterol run in the family? I suppose you may want to brace yourself for the likely heart disease that may spell your doom one day. What about that creative gene that you so desperately wish you had? If only the gods had been gracious enough to imbed that code in you since your parents just didn't seem to have it wired in them to pass down to you. Or maybe you were cursed with the dreaded fat gene. Guess it just means you are doomed to live on diets and pills the rest of your life. These old beliefs are now beginning to be challenged and even shattered with new discoveries involving epigenetics.

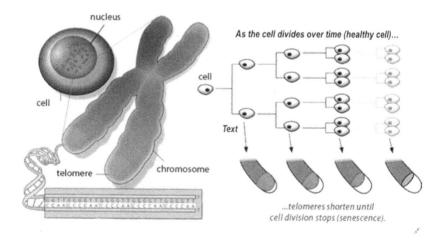

...telomeres shorten until cell division stops (senescence).

Epigenetics is the study of how our lives and environment cause levels of interactions within our genes. Scientists are learning that the genes we have at birth do not determine the complete outcome of our futures. Essentially—through our focus, lifestyle, health, and meditation—we can affect changes in our cells regarding how they read information from our genes, thus generating changes within our body. That's right. We are not wired and set for life at birth. We have the ability to change the deck of cards we were dealt from our parents.

Telo Me More

To begin understanding how this works, we first must understand the terminology behind telomeres and telomerase, along with their responsibilities in our genes. Telomeres are the protective DNA-protein structures that are located at the ends of our chromosomes. As we age, we find that these telomeres shrink in size, resulting in cellular breakdown. Telomerase is the ribonucleoprotein that replenishes the DNA within the telomeres. If enough telomerase is available, it counters the progressive shorting of our telomeres on our chromosomes that would normally occur as we age. In short, we slow down the aging progress with telomerase. We can stave off gray hair, wrinkles, crow's feet, and varicose veins.

Ever wonder how or why some people just look younger than their age without plastic surgery? Whether they realize it or not, they likely have more telomerase in their systems helping their bodies stay younger. This gives new meaning to "age is just a number."

Quick return to eighth grade biology: what do all cells need for creation? Protein. How do they get this protein? It comes from our DNA and chromosomes. Decades ago, it was taught and believed that our DNA provides this protein, but what has been discovered is actually different. When new cell growth happens, a signal is sent out to our DNA that causes the protective sleeve covering our chromosomes to be lifted. Once the original DNA (blueprint) is exposed, a protein known as RNA polymerase binds to the exposed DNA gene, moves down the length of that gene, and makes an RNA copy of the gene. So, what does the actual gene do? Nothing—it is just a blueprint. What gives our cells and bodies the signals they need to conduct this activity? It is the process of epigenetics. Older conventional teachings taught that DNA converts to RNA and then into protein for our cells. It has turned the teachings of the previous fifty years upside down that our genes are programing the proteins that make up our cellular structures. It is the RNA copy of the DNA that goes out into the cell in order to manufacture proteins that generate new cells.

Epigenetics is the process of changing the readout of the original gene. Not changing the original blueprint or genes themselves, but the copy that goes into our new cells being produced. What has been discovered is that we can change the signals that conduct the epigenetics process.

Ultimately, we are not our genes. We change the readouts by our environments and through our perceptions of our environments. Through this process, we can slow the effects of aging through the impact we put on our cells. Once again, this comes down to the mind and what thought energy we are placing in our bodies. With less stress and damage to our cells, we can keep more telomerase in our cells, thus slowing down the aging of the cells, and live a more prolonged, healthy life. Do you want to look like sixty when you are eighty? This is how it begins.

Thoughts on Cancer

In 2008 a study from the Proceedings of the National Academy of Sciences (PNAS) was published concerning the lifestyle changes in men and how those changes could modify the progression of prostate cancer. The study involved thirty men with low-risk prostate cancers who aged in range from 49–80 years old. Eighty-four percent of the men identified their ethnicity as Caucasian, 9% Hispanic, 3% Asian, and 4% African American. Two-thirds of the men were married, and 72% were employed at the time. These men did not undergo any radiation treatment or surgery for their low-risk tumors; instead, they were assigned in-depth lifestyle changes such as low-fat whole foods, plant-based nutrition, stress management, moderate exercise, and participation within a psychosocial support group. Their gene expression composites of all their prostates were copied before the test period began. For all prescriptions they were on, those dosages were kept the same. The test was to last ninety days.

At the conclusion of the test period, a significant improvement in cardiovascular health was noted including lowered blood pressure. Waist circumference decreased along with a reported decrease in psychological distress along with an increase in mental and cognitive competency. The final testing showed 48 upregulated and 453 downregulated transcripts in normal prostate tissue after 3 months of intervention; meaning that nearly 87% of the cancer tissues in the prostate decreased.

Is there a gene we have that causes cancer? I am not of that mindset. It is my belief that cancer cells grow within us when we are under stress, anxiety, and living out of balance with the natural harmony of the earth. We begin to send signals to our cells that, like us, are out of balance. I believe it is this unbalancing of sorts that may allow cancer cells to grow within us.

We must recognize what it means to be out of balance with what the Universe has provided for us. Yes, it comes down to our immediate environment and what we subject ourselves to each day regarding mental and physical stressors, but it is also very much about what we allow ourselves to consume for nutrition. I'm not advocating forbidding ourselves to live a life worth enjoying food and drink, but rather to always understand what it means to consume with moderation.

Taking Action on Knowledge

After the readings I came across involving the connection of lifestyle and cellular impact, I made some conscious decisions to change areas of my life. I cut out soda completely from my diet as well as all fried foods and most meat. I live now as a pescatarian (fish eater, but no other meats) and consume a mostly plant-based diet. I stopped finding excuses not to exercise each day and committed to a forty-five-minute workout regimen each morning without fail. I decided I would never take a day off despite what advice may be given from the physical exercise experts. My exercise routine is a mostly cardio regimen and typically a low-impact one. I figured my then-thirty-nine-year-old body could handle it and recover daily without the need for a day off.

It is a forty-five-minute indoor bike, or a four-mile run outside on my favorite trail; regardless of which, I did it religiously for an entire year (as of this writing, I am nearing two years and don't intend to change my routine). I lost nearly 60 pounds in 6 months transforming my body from 250 pounds down to 190. I'm not completely perfect in my daily routine, as I allow myself to succumb to tantalizing temptations such as a piece of cheesecake or my other Achille's heel: peanut butter and chocolate. The point is no one needs to be perfect but to simply stay committed to the routine.

> Knowledge is not power. It is simply potential power depending on the choice to take action or not.

I don't know what my gene expression was before my yearlong commitment, but I know it was heading down a dark road with a dead-end had I not made the changes to my environment, attitude, and perceptions. When I went to have my routine six-month blood work with my doctor, he told me he'd likely not see anyone the rest of the year with cholesterol levels better than mine. This came from a man who at one time had to have his nurse frantically call me to report a test readout of 300+, fearful if I didn't get on medication quickly, my heart would explode.

The Inner Voice

Even though science has been slow to validate some of the understandings expressed in the above sections, it is becoming clearer that where our attention goes, energy flows. What we think literally generates our outcomes. We need to be very mindful of the voice inside our heads. Do any of these thoughts sound familiar to you?

- I'm always tired.
- I don't have time for exercise.
- Working out is too hard.
- I can't ever get enough sleep.
- I'm just a weak and sick person—always have been and always will be.
- I can't quit sugar—I love it too much.
- I can't quit fried foods when I travel for work as much as I do.
- I'm too old.
- My mind just isn't what it used to be.

These are the types of limiting programs we continue to run in the background and often don't realize impact us in negative ways.

Think of the challenges and struggles you may be facing in life. Whatever area they may be in, you likely have a list like this too. It may vary based on the area of focus, but most people walk around every day programming their bodies via their thoughts—most of which are limiting and negative.

Think of how these beliefs are serving you and how they are not. Think about how they are healing you or harming you. In most cases, you will find that your inner voice is harming you each day. Slowly, and over the course of your lifetime, that chatter in your head is programming the connection to the cells in your body—literally telling and feeding them the commands from your head.

In order to make the positive changes, we need to rewrite the code being sent to our bodies. We know that positive thoughts can make us happier, and negative thoughts often make us sadder. Why don't we think in the same terminology around how our thoughts impact our health? Our own thoughts can make us weaker or sicker—as well as stronger and more immune.

These new and miraculous discoveries are showing us the truth that gene expression can and will be influenced by our environments and daily activity. It also lays out hopeful foundations for similar breakthroughs with different types of cancers such as colon cancer and breast cancer.

Once we have the knowledge and the proof of these types of truths, it really does all come down to a choice and personal commitment. We need to get out of our own way and stop with the excuses we generate for why we need to have that greasy burger or down all those sugary soft drinks. These delicacies are often out of balance with what the Universe has already provided for us. It is not that we must do away completely with the things we love in life; it is just becoming more aware of keeping ourselves within balance that very well may make all the difference between living in sync or out of sync with life. Each has its rewards as well as its punishments.

We have the choice through every moment of every day. Let's commit to the Ungraduation process each day to begin to think ourselves well. Once you begin this healthy thinking, the actions soon follow. We cannot think ourselves healthy and also take part in poor diet habits. It all works in unison. I promise you that when you begin the practice, you'll see massive rewards in health, body, and mind.

Ungraduated Call to Action

- Start with daily positive affirmation such as, "I am healthy, my body is strong, and my cells are full of growth and vitality." Write this or say this to yourself five times in the morning and evening.

- Take action and begin an exercise routine. It can start with ten minutes a day, and you can build from there. Make it something you enjoy doing, and do it every day.
- Make a list of all the inner voice beliefs you have about your body and age. Then write next to those things what you want to change about yourself, and keep that list in a prominent location every day. Refer to and read that list beginning each day to start rewiring your old beliefs about your body.
- Track your weight, health, and overall mental fitness for three months. You will begin to notice a difference.

Chapter 9
Manifest Your Life

"Accept what comes to you woven in the pattern of your destiny, for what could more aptly fit your needs?"
~ Marcus Aurelius ~

It was 2012, and I could feel a big change was coming in my life even though a big change had already occurred. I had been promoted from the level of Area Supervisor responsible for ten restaurants to Director of Operations having the responsibility for around sixty restaurants. That was already a big shift, but life still had more plans of change in store for me. My wife and I had been living in eastern Pennsylvania at the time, and I knew that it would not be long before it would be time for another move. We had already moved from Pittsburgh, PA, to Tampa, FL, and from Tampa to the Philadelphia area. Ever since leaving the rolling hills of western Pennsylvania, my wife and I had expressed a desire to be back closer to our families in the Pittsburgh area.

Shortly after my change in position, my promoting supervisor left the company. His predecessor, my new boss, came to me in a matter of weeks, asking me if I would consider another move.

"Depends on where it is," I said to him.

"We have two options for you. Either you can move back to your hometown of Pittsburgh, Pennsylvania, and be responsible for operations there, or we have an opening to run the Cleveland, Ohio, market. It's your choice."

I could barely wait to tell my wife the great news. While we were enjoying our lives in eastern Pennsylvania, we knew we both wanted to get closer to home. The better opportunity at the time seemed to be the Cleveland market. Sales were higher in that part of the country than Pittsburgh, and while both markets represented great opportunities, I settled on Cleveland. My wife and I began looking at areas to live that would be close enough to Pittsburgh to be near family, but also within Ohio, so I could live within my new territory.

The Synchronicities of Manifestation

In 2013, the real-estate market was still mostly in recovery mode from the Great Recession. We had barely escaped Florida and the housing market there ahead of the crash. One of the most overinflated housing markets at the time was in Florida. We were paying far too much for our home mortgage with the ballooning real estate market prerecession. We were fortunate to almost break even on our move to Pennsylvania. Had we not gotten out of Florida in 2007, and made the move to Pennsylvania, we would have been so upside down on our mortgage that we may have been forced into foreclosure in the months and years that ensued due to real estate and financial crises from 2008 through 2011.

We were facing a move to Ohio in 2013, and the market was still quite shaky. Banks had learned their lessons and were becoming far stricter in whom they approved for home loans. The company's request for me was to move as quickly as I possibly could. So after only nine months in my new position, we sought out a real estate agent and began the arduous task of putting our house on the market.

After the first meeting with our new agent and agreeing on what would be a fair but aggressive listing price to spur as much attention as we could in what was a cautious real estate market, we decided to list at the exact price we needed to be able to pay off the mortgage.

Even though we had lived there from 2007 to 2013, the market hadn't gained enough value to net us any equity in our home. It would be far more likely with listing at the starting price that we needed to break even that we'd get lowball offers from ambitious buyers looking to take full advantage of a buyer's market. We weren't even sure if we'd be able to afford the move if we didn't get a decent enough offer to get out of our home in Pennsylvania. The circumstances and events that transpired still are nothing short of awe-inspiring and amazing to me.

Here we go.

Upon our signing the contract with our new real estate agent, he proceeded outside to begin putting the for-sale sign in the yard. Anyone who has ever sold a home knows this moment. It's the point in time that all the neighbors begin to get a bit nosier and also the point in time you begin to become more self-reflective. Seeing the for-sale sign in the ground is a point of finite endings as well as hopeful new beginnings.

As I stood there half watching him and reflecting on my life in that home, he began pounding the sign in and securing it in place. I couldn't help wondering what would happen next. I noticed a car coming around the bend in our street and slowing down. They rolled their window down and started a conversation with our new agent.

As he looked away from the couple in the car and back toward the house, I saw him make a gesture toward me to come out.

I opened the door and walked to the curb.

He proceeded to ask me if it would be OK to allow this couple to view our home. He told us they were from the New York City area and looking for a quieter place to retire and call home. They were only there for the weekend, and upon seeing our for-sale sign go in the ground, wanted to know if they could take a look at the house.

In my mind I was thinking, *Hmmm—this is rather random. What are the chances of a car just happening to pass by at the exact time that our for-sale sign was going in the ground?*

Now in most situations, my wife would freak out and say, "No way—there isn't anyone coming into this house before I've had the chance to make it presentable." She has always taken great pride in showing our home in the best light possible, and I've always appreciated this about her. But the situation was unique. We each knew every showing would matter with a market that was going to be less favorable to us. So, we let them see the house along with some requests for grace since we hadn't had the time to get the house ready to show.

My wife and I walked across the street to our good friends and neighbors and sat down with them on their porch while our strangely timed visitors were walking through our home.

I remember it taking far longer than I anticipated. I assumed it could be a good sign. If buyers exit too quickly, it usually means signs of disinterest. Anxiously, I tried to enjoy a beer with my friend and neighbor on that very atypical Sunday afternoon. I had enjoyed many good adult beverages on that porch while looking at my home, but that moment was far different—and I felt it.

Trying to Get "Stuck in Ohio"

As the couple from New York exited the home, I saw them shake hands with our new agent, get back into their car, and pull out of the driveway. My wife and I made our way back over toward our home and noticed a glowing smile coming from Jack, our agent. "They made you guys an offer," he said.

Already flabbergasted, I completely expected to hear a lowball offer. "Their offer is exactly at the listing price, with one condition . . . the theatre room your wife and her dad built in the basement stays as-is." The look on my face had to show my astonishment. Here was the first viewing of my home, which only occurred because of the exact moment our agent was putting a sign in the ground, when a couple that just happened to be in town were looking for a retirement home in my community. Coincidence? I think not.

The story gets better from here. My wife and I had already planned a trip to Ohio the following weekend to begin our own house-hunting expedition. We fully expected to be taking that trip with only the ability to look at homes and not able to make offers. No agents would take a serious offer from a homebuyer who was currently locked into a mortgage. Receiving the offer enabled us to get a letter from our bank that stated we had a buyer locked in to purchase our home. Contingent on our buyers coming through, we could make a serious offer if we found a home we liked in Ohio. We had their offer locked in, and if they backed out for any reason, we would keep their down payment, making it unlikely for them to want to back out. With a letter and statement of good faith from our buyers in hand, we drove to Ohio to meet our agent there.

We had a less-than-fruitful experience through most of the homes we were shown. Nothing fit our expectations, and we were beginning to wonder if we'd even have a place to live in Ohio once our home sold since we had already agreed to vacate our old house by a certain date.

The weekend was dying down and in a less-than-enthusiastic voice, our agent began telling us of another option within our price range that had been on the market for some time. She passed the printouts and pictures to me, and as I flipped through them, my instinct was to tell her to skip it. There seemed to be far too much old wallpaper and dated look to the home. It felt just like all the others we had seen to that point.

She must have seen the disappointment on my face, asking, "It's just right up the road; are you sure you don't want to see it?"

I was about to say let's keep going past it, but my wife said, "What the heck. Let's just at least drive past it and see."

As we pulled up, the charm of the house caught our eye. Once inside, my wife and I expressed our love for the character and bones of the house and how the pictures just didn't do it justice. We probably spent two hours plus walking that home, and when our time there had come to an end, we were telling our agent we wanted to make an offer.

Knowing we had just received the good fortune of not receiving a lowball buyer's market offer from the people who were buying our home in Pennsylvania, we decided to make a fair offer on the house in Ohio. We made them an offer that was only $10,000 less than their asking price, telling our agent to convey to their agent that we love the home, but it will require some work and upgrades. Then we crossed our fingers while our agent called their agent to give them the news. My wife and I had decided to go to dinner, and as the hours passed, we worked to keep our hopes up as much as we could.

The phone rang. It was our agent, and she had called to tell us our offer had been accepted. All we would need to do was put down a $5,000 good-faith payment to lock in the offer, just as the buyers for our home had done. There was one problem. We hadn't brought our checkbook. I remember looking at my wife like it was her fault. After all, she was the far more responsible one who was supposed to think of things like this.

It was Sunday afternoon, and banks were closed. Even if we had found an open bank, our bank did not have a branch in Ohio. We would have no way to take out $5,000 unless we drove back home the seven hours and were able to wire the money. Our agent politely informed us that any offer that would come in to the sellers of the home would be fair game. We wouldn't be able to hold our place without the $5,000 good-faith down payment.

We were finishing our dinner at a place called The Magic Tree Pub & Brewery. My wife rather frantically began digging through her purse. Since she handled all the finances for us, she was hoping somehow, some way, she may have brought her checkbook. She dug and dug but to no avail.

Then, a smile arose on her face, and she slowly pulled out a crumpled-up piece of yellowish paper. She straightened it out and held it for me to see. "Here's our ticket," she said. In her purse was one random, folded-up, discarded, forgotten-about check. How and why it was there when we had forgotten our checkbook was just another example of life manifesting its synchronicity when you least expect it but most need it.

We called our agent and told her we'd meet her to give her the check and make our offer final.

Could this have been a random event? Sure, I suppose so. But the events leading up to it from how our house sold in Pennsylvania, to how we almost skipped the house in Ohio due to it not looking good in the pictures, and then to randomly finding one folded-up check in a purse so we could make an offer on a new home? Too many coincidences for me. And this is just one of the many examples and stories I could have told that have unfolded in my life. Chances are you have many of these stories, too.

Being able to land this dream home enabled me to get to Ohio quickly and begin the next chapter of my career. It allowed me to be in the best place for my business and the ability to be near my family. Had I not found this specific home, what would be different? I'm honestly not sure, but I know this—this was the home we were meant to be in, and we both knew it. Apparently, the Universe agreed and helped make it happen.

Life Is not Random

The Universal Principles and Laws discussed in chapter three are always in effect whether we realize it or not. The Universe is providing for us daily, yet most are completely unaware of the signals we receive from beyond our awareness. Each of us is generating our own reality, but most tend to be asleep at the wheel of life. How can we grab hold of the steering wheel and take full advantage of what the Universe is offering us? We start by paying attention to what is placed in front of us. I can say from experience, we get back what we put out into the Universe with thought. Sometimes this happens instantaneously, yet other times it may take a few days, weeks, or months—depending on the intentions we broadcast. Just know this: we will get back what we put out.

The Field of Potentiality

The field of potentiality is always open for business. Envision a bright neon sign flashing "Open 24 Hours." That is the gateway to all our limitations as well as vast amounts of greatest potential.

Whether we like to acknowledge it or not, the field of potentiality is always listening to our thoughts. We can hide nothing from it. It hears us when we are at our best and at our worst. Over time, we become the product of those thoughts. Every present moment, we forge our futures of potential. Will we generate futures of prosperity and fulfillment or of regret and negativity? The choice is up to us.

Not many years ago, I read *E-Squared* by Pam Grout. The book is all about the field of potentiality and how we can test this field through some basic DIY-type experiments. I devoured the material and decided I would put my own manifesting abilities to the test through some of the experiments. The only key to the successful outcomes was to meditate intently on the desired outcome with exact expectations and timeframes for the outcomes. The intentions had to be specific, without any room for misinterpretation or coincidence.

Here is one real-life example from my own experience. I sat quietly one evening before dinner. I closed my eyes and focused my mind with great intention. I put out to the Universe with all my might, focus, and belief that I wanted to receive some gift of monetary value. I was sure to let the Universe know that it needed not be of any massive value, I just simply wanted to know that this capability was possible. I focused the thought that it must be unique and undeniable. For example, I couldn't simply be walking down the street and stumble across a shiny penny—no, it must be a far greater proof of reality.

I held this intention in my mind for about twenty minutes, making sure all the while that I told myself I would receive my validation within exactly three days. That was my deadline. Upon the completion of this silent meditation, I thanked the Universe mentally for listening and granting my request. I walked away from the moment already knowing without a doubt in my mind that I would receive my answer and gift. My only job was to pay attention to what the Universe was going to place in front of me.

I made sure to leave no stone unturned over those next three days, looking for my gift from the Universe. I experienced a couple possibilities but remembered my request of the Universe that it had to be unique, meaning the gift couldn't come through work, my family, or close friends. It had to come from some very unexpected, outside-of-the-norm place or interaction. As the days wore on, all the while, I kept in my mind the knowing that I would indeed receive the gift. Never once doubting that I would get my answer, I received it almost exactly 72 hours later when my cell phone rang.

Looking down at my phone, I saw that it was a local number, but I did not recognize it. Like most others do with telephone numbers we don't recognize, I let the call go to voicemail. After a minute or so, I listened to that message. The message went something like this: "Hello, Ken. This is _____ from Things Remembered. We can see in our records that you haven't visited us in a while, and we're calling to inform you that you have a $50 store credit as a gift to use at your convenience. We value your business and hope that this gift brings you in to see us again soon."

If anyone had seen me in that moment . . . I must have had that dazed and confused look of absolute bewilderment. I sat there, mouth agape, absolutely shocked. I had *never* received a call before, out of blue and completely randomly, from a department store telling me that they were deciding to issue me a store credit. I hadn't returned anything to them, had not reached out to them, was not waiting for or aware of any type of promotions they were running for past customers, and yet I had received that phone call at nearly the exact point at which I had, with intention, given to the Universe (field of potentiality) as my deadline just three days earlier. I didn't receive this message as an email. It wasn't a random coupon or voucher sent to me through the mail. No, it was a phone call, from some store employee—letting me know that they decided to issue me $50 to come and spend at my leisure.

Instantly I knew it was my sign from the Universe. It fit every specific point I had asked for as a sign that this manifesting stuff is real. I needed something so unique and specific, and I had received it right as intended. Did I mention the store name? Things Remembered. That seemed to be a little twist of irony and humor from the Universe itself, as if to say—yup, I remembered. Mind blown.

As if that wasn't enough, I decided I would put my newfound powers to the absolute test and try some more in-the-moment possibilities. After I had energetically finished telling my wife what just happened, we went out to our back deck in our Ohio home, where I often take in the beauty of nature and brilliance of life. I'm fortunate enough to have an array of wildlife I can watch and catch glimpses of as I wonder off into thought. That time, however, I was intent on using some manifesting abilities to see if I could actually will some wildlife before my eyes.

In my backyard, it is not uncommon to see chipmunks, squirrels, and many different types of birds. Chipmunks and squirrels were some of my favorites to observe as they went about their habitual search of nuts, berries, and other meals while scurrying about. As I sat there, I put out the intention that I would like to see a rabbit. I had seen rabbits before in my backyard but far less commonly. I told myself I would like to now see a rabbit come into my view. Once again, I believed it with all my heart that this would happen. I left no room for any other possibility in my mind. It simply was going to happen. I sat there, eyes open that time, but just intently focused on the nature scene in front of me waiting to see the rabbit that I knew was going to creep into my vision. There had been no rabbit sighting for quite some time; weeks at least. But in that moment, I was calling out to it—any rabbit, for that matter. Just come on out and join the frolicking of its wildlife friends.

I knew my wife may have had some trepidations about my beliefs and experiments, but she was about to witness at least some small glimpse of the power of manifestation. After about twenty minutes, I had closed my eyes and was just allowing the warm sunlight to kiss my face while taking in the beautiful sounds of the scene around me.

"Kenny..." (only she and my mother call me Kenny, by the way) she whispered from my side. "Look." She gestured toward the right of our backyard, where this little gray bunny had slowly hopped into our view.

I felt a sudden rush of energy as the Universe basically said to me, "Here you go. Ask and you shall receive." Tears began welling up in my eyes. I'm not someone that typically cries over seeing bunny rabbits. Those were complete tears of joy from beginning to understand, and no longer simply hoping or believing, that we have an ability to influence our realities. These experiences were teaching and showing me proof and the validation that I needed that we influence our lives from a place of true inner power. Those were some examples of my own simple manifestations. Those were just a few of my own personal validations from the Universe I needed to cement the fact that we are indeed bringing into our lives each day what we think and put out into the field of potentiality.

This is the Law of Correspondence at work. As above, so below. As we put out thought into the energy field of life and the Universe, we get back those thoughts, some sooner than others, but we always get those thoughts back.

What Thoughts Are You Manifesting?

Really stop and think about this. What type of thoughts are you putting out into the field of potentiality each day? Are they thoughts of empowerment? Or are they self-deprecating thoughts, such as "I'm not good enough" or "I'm not deserving"? Think of the negative thoughts that we consciously tell ourselves. It's no wonder with the number of limiting beliefs we tell ourselves each day that our subconscious and unconscious minds take over and often give us back exactly what we are putting out—limitations.

To change our realities for the better, we must become aware of the thoughts we exude. We are not our thoughts, but we will become them. That is the perspective that is powerful to understand. The Universe is always listening and granting you what you give it—it doesn't judge whether it is good or bad for you. It simply gives unconditionally.

What side of the giving do you want to manifest? Start with becoming aware of your thoughts. We all are always manifesting our realities through every waking and ever-present moment. What will your reality look like in one month, one year, or five years? Pay attention to your thoughts—they are your crystal ball to your future self and woven into your pattern of future destiny.

Ungraduated Call to Action

- Try your own manifesting test—meditate on something specific for twenty minutes following these guidelines:
    1. Exact thing you expect or want
    2. By when (exact date and time—three days to a week is fair game)
    3. Has to be a clear sign (make it unequivocally unique)
    4. *Believe* it to be with all your heart, leaving no doubt in your mind that you'll receive it (any small doubt puts that signal out and you may miss your sign)

- What limiting beliefs are you broadcasting to the Universe each day? Write these down, and then write their exact opposite. Work to reprogram your mind to think the positive opposites of what you are thinking about yourself. Document your progress for thirty days.

Part 4
Taking Action & Living Your Purpose

Chapter 10

The Power of Belief

"The outer conditions of a person's life will always be found to reflect their inner beliefs."
~ James Allen ~

Jean-Dominique Bauby was a French editor-in-chief of a well-known magazine, *Elle*, as well as an actor and author. He lived a large and fulfilling life. In 1995, Jean-Do, as he was widely known, was enjoying a drive with his son when he suddenly began experiencing double vision. He was rushed to a hospital, where he slipped into a coma and remained in intensive care for three weeks.

Upon Jean-Do's awakening, he was paralyzed from head to toe and diagnosed with a rare condition known as locked-in syndrome, resulting from a stroke. At the age of forty-three, his life would be completely changed. He could no longer eat or breathe without assistance. His prognosis wasn't good. Even though he could still feel his body, he wasn't able to move anything except his left eyelid, which he could blink.

One day while sitting in the hospital with Jean-Do, Bernard Chapuis, former editor of *Men's Vogue* and friend of Jean-Do, noticed the twitching and blinking of his left eye. Bernard asked Jean-Do if he could understand him, and if so, to blink his eye. Jean-Do responded in the affirmative with a blink of an eye.

What transpired next resulted in Jean-Do spending months learning a skill known as the alphabet of silence. His therapist would call out and point to letters most frequently used in the

French language, and Jean-Do would make words and phrases by blinking his eye upon receiving the letter he wanted to use.

What manifested from this translation of letters and blinks of an eye was a bestselling memoir titled *The Diving Bell and the Butterfly*. It took Jean-Do 200,000 blinks to write the story about what it was like to be trapped inside of his own body. The book's title refers to the immobility of his body by comparing it to old-fashioned heavy diving headgear. Meanwhile, inside he describes his mind fluttering as delicately as a butterfly. Later, Jean-Do's book was turned into a critically acclaimed movie that has been nominated for four Academy Awards.

Through the help and assistance of his specialized nurse, Claude Mendibil, Jean-Do was able to write his book. Mendibil spent three hours, six days a week, taking dictation from Jean-Do by using the same method he was taught by his speech therapist. Each night, he would review and memorize his thoughts so that when Mendibil arrived the next day to dictate for him, he could transcribe the latest installments to his book.

What would most of us have done if faced with that grim outlook and diagnosis? Would we have had the belief that we could communicate and still deliver on our life goals? Would we dig deep, decide what we still had control over in life, and find a way to persevere? This is a difficult scenario for anyone to try to envision, but all too often, life throws misfortune into the lives of many. It is how we respond in any given scenario that determines our outcomes.

> If you have been programming your belief that money is evil and you should not have more than you need, then this is exactly what you are bringing into your life: lack of money.

Fortunately for many, we are not faced with these challenges. We have the power of thought and belief on our side, but so often we don't realize the gold mine we are standing on. Many of us walk around blinded by fear, preprogrammed beliefs from family or social belief systems given to us through our jobs, media, and friends. We allow these mostly limiting beliefs to keep hidden far from our awareness the keys to the treasure.

Unconscious Self-Talk

There is such a thing as *unconscious self-talk*. This self-talk occurs under the surface of our conscious awareness and plays itself out in the part of our minds that operates without thought in a subconscious manner. The overlying programs that we tell ourselves and others are always running on autopilot in the background of our minds. Let's think of some other examples of labels we give ourselves each day whether we realize it or not.

Assume for a moment that you label yourself in your mind's eye as fat or stupid. You may not come out with those descriptors to someone asking you about yourself, but the simple act of thinking it puts that thought form energy out into the field, and it is then bounced back to us in a program that says: "OK—you wish to be 'fat' or 'stupid.'"

The Universal field of energy that we are interacting with on a continual never-ending basis while we are alive is very literal. It is going to give you back everything that you place out into it.

Do you live a life fearful of change? That is what you get back—fear of anything that does not stay constant in your life. Do you constantly find yourself yearning and desiring more money? The Universal Field says, "OK, you don't have enough money—I'll be sure to keep it that way for you."

Are you someone who is always wondering why you keep finding yourself in hurtful and bad relationships? It is very likely the thought energy being emitted from you into the field is asking to continue to give you the same type of relationships that you have been getting. It may sound like this: "I can't ever seem to find a loving, respectful partner with whom I can see myself in a mutual and loving relationship." Do you see the flaw of that thought? You get back exactly what you put out—"as above, so below"—again, as explained by the Principle of Correspondence.

The key here to crack the code is simple. We've all heard of positive affirmations. They are good, but we must be careful in terms of the specificity through which we engage with them. For example, an affirmation that says, "I will be happy and prosperous." Sounds good right? But you can see the subtle future tense of "I *will*." That needs to be in the present tense—"I *am* happy and prosperous." Every thought needs to be manifested in the present tense, in *the now*. We need to envision ourselves already having the experience. *That is key*. That is what positive self-affirmations are all about and how we manifest our highest potential.

Another key component of this thinking is coming to the very truth of how powerful we are. If you are the type of person who sits around each day thinking about how insignificant and small you are, that is exactly what you will remain. The literalness of the Universal Field of energy will ensure it. No matter how we view ourselves in the grand scheme of life and manmade labels, we must learn to understand we are all-encompassing, all-powerful creators of life and reality. Our thoughts really are the power that forms our lives. Put this reality out into the field instead: "I am powerful and free of boundaries—I attain anything that I desire, now. I am with immense abundance."

What we resist persists. If we fight for our limitations, we get to keep them. "I can't—I'm not good enough." Our brains are like supercomputers that run the programs of thought form energy. We are always getting back what we put out. Self-talk is the program that runs our brain and its communication with our body.

Belief Knows no Boundaries

In Viktor E. Frankl's amazing book *Man's Search for Meaning*, there may be no better story for why we need to be aware of our power of belief. Viktor was arrested during the Holocaust, placed into Jewish concentration camps, and tortured both mentally and physically. Others didn't live beyond a few weeks or months, but Viktor survived three years in Auschwitz and Dachau. Viktor is quoted in his book by stating, "Everything can be taken from a man but one thing—the last of the human freedoms—to choose one's attitude in any given set of circumstances, to choose one's own way."[22]

In his book, he speaks to being able to generate the mindset and will to live that superseded the horrendous physical treatment, starvation, and mental torture he received. Because he envisioned himself surviving and having a purpose to tell his story and hoped to see his loved ones again—he painted a mental frame of reference that allowed his positive mental state to endure, which enabled him to persevere and survive. That was the one thing his captors couldn't strip him of.

There are times that we forge the mental image of achievement to accomplish goals, and then there are times that different levels of authority dictate that belief to us. These varying levels of belief play out in our society every day. We often don't pause to consider the powerful evidence that exists in terms of our belief system and what it does for programming the mind and thus the body.

Our minds are tools that can be used for empowerment and freedom or for mental and physical slavery and even death. If there were a drug available for this type of amazing effect on the open market, what would it sell for? We have this innate power within us, yet so few have the ability to recognize it.

The Origin of Belief

According to Kundalini Master Santosh Sachdeva, "A belief is nothing more than a generalization of a past incident." At early ages, our experiences are downloaded from our families, friends, and the organizations in which we take part. They help mold our view of the world around us. Everything in our world as children and young adults comes from our surroundings and experiences. Unless we were any different from others, we accepted these viewpoints and belief systems. It isn't until we begin to mature that we begin to challenge our own views of ourselves and the world around us. However, whether most of us realize it or not, much of how we view the world has been hardwired into us by the time we are ten years old. From the beliefs of others, we are taught what to think and feel about many things:

> What mental state are you mostly in each day? Really look at this. It answers how life works with you or against you.

- Whom to trust and not trust
- What good and bad relationships are
- Which emotions are good and bad
- What's possible and not possible
- What is of value and not of value
- What is right and wrong

It is through these thoughts and belief systems that we learn to form our core belief systems about who we are as well as others in the world around us:

- The world is safe / the world is dangerous.
- Life has meaning, order, and purpose / life is random.
- People are basically well intended / people are basically ill intended.
- Most people are trustworthy / most people are untrustworthy.
- I generate my own outcomes / I am controlled by fate and have no impact on my life.
- I am competent and strong / I am vulnerable and weak.
- Life flows and is satisfying / Life is a constant struggle and an uphill battle.

- Work is about fulfillment / Work is a necessary means to earn money.

Each of these belief systems spawns hundreds of other beliefs. The question we need to ask ourselves is how much of these preprogrammed beliefs downloaded from society and our upbringing do we choose to reflect us now? What do we ultimately want to be, and how should we view the world through our own eyes?

Even though beliefs are not facts, we often live with them as if they are. This is due to how our beliefs become connected to our emotions and memories. It is a sort of fusing of belief systems that becomes solidified in us. Until we explore the deeper meaning of our own beliefs, they often run on autopilot. The main point to understand is this: our beliefs either empower us or limit us. The choice is up to us.

While many of the beliefs instilled in us during our early years served us at the time, some of these beliefs are habitual programs we run. They steal our energy and keep us in undesirable situations due to their negative outcomes. While it is not easy to remove old limiting life beliefs, it is certainly possible.

The power of belief is always a powerful tool and one that we need to keep in mind as we face life's challenges. While many of us will face obstacles (small and large) the attitude and way in which we frame them will decide how we come through them on the other end. The fact that all thought creates form on some level can be a difficult perspective to wrap your mind around. Many have heard the phrase, "I think, therefore I am." What this means is exactly what it states. As we move through time, our thoughts create our reality. All thought is form on some level, meaning that if you think it enough, you manifest it into your reality. There truly are no idle thoughts or beliefs.

Be mindful of your thoughts and self-talk. You are literally thinking your life into existence each moment of every day. While we never wish to find ourselves in situations like that of Jean-Dominique Bauby or Viktor Frankl, we can choose our mental mindset and belief system—in good times and in those that are more challenging.

Beliefs on Money

Money—the root of all evil, or so it has often been coined. Humankind created money for a variety of reasons. A farmer needed a pair of shoes from the shoemaker, and the shoemaker in turn needed corn to feed his family. The barter system worked, but as more needs grew through time and our nomadic lifestyle transitioned across geographies, humans needed a more efficient system with which to transact. The farmer simply couldn't take all his crops with him wherever he went in order to be able to exchange for other goods or services. A shoemaker wasn't easily able to generate a stockpile of shoes to travel around with in hopes that he'd come across people who needed them. Thus, the first currency was created.

Coins of all types were created so that transactions could be made easier for all parties. These first currencies date all the way back to the days of the Mayans, Incas, and many other ancient civilizations. Eventually Europeans began defining gold and other precious metals as money.

Society eventually made its way to paper promissory notes that were backed by gold at one time.

Today, currency is quantified by nothing more than digits on a computer screen. It's quite humorous to me in the present era how not enough actual paper money exists to support the amounts that sit as digital icons in the bank accounts across the globe. We have come to a point of fantasy with money. So much so that the world runs in such a way that there isn't enough real money to go around, so we operate on "trust" of a particular "government-backed" dollar bill—nothing more. The government keeps the system chugging along around the world. Everything is pinned in price to the

US Dollar. Anyone who reads this can make their own conclusions on how "real" money is or isn't.

The late great author and writer Shakti Gawain is quoted in her book *Living in the Light* as saying, "If you are denying money, you are also denying a big part of the energy of the Universe and the way the world works." The book gives many great perspectives on how to embrace life and live positively through intuition and how to try to address the many challenges and questions that come into existence in many of our lives. One of which is money.

If you have always operated on a survival level with money, having only enough money to take care of your basic needs, that's where your money will go. If you start to attract more money into your life, you may have the tendency to increase your basic needs and still only make enough to survive. Could money or the lack thereof all really be about *mindset*? I believe so. Like so many other things in life, you have to ask yourself a key question. *Are you worth it?* The answer is simply yes. We are all worthy of living an exceptional life with enough money to provide for ourselves and others.

Back to chapter three and Universal Law, this perspective ties back to the Principle of Mentalism. Money has as much to do with thought and belief as anything else we have discussed. If you have been programming yourself that "money is evil," and "I should not have more than I need," then this very well may be what you are bringing into your life with your thoughts. If this is the case, then how can you make the biggest difference for others in the world if that is the mental construct you choose to believe? Most of us know that money doesn't buy happiness. Those who have more money than they know what to do with will admit this if they are honest. Humanity at its core craves purpose. And when you have purpose, money can help you achieve purpose. More often than not, this is the case.

Whether we like it or not, the world runs on money. I personally wish the world operated on a sort of merit system, of which we simply did what we are skilled at for the betterment of all society, but those types of utopian dreams are simply that, at least for now. So rather than wish and hope for change, or shun money, why not try to change our mindset on the topic? Why not say we *do deserve* to make more of this thing the world runs on, so that we can help in the best ways possible for our own needs and the needs of others?

Just putting it out there—perhaps money is what you make of it. Just like the rest of the physical world we live in. *Think and Grow Rich* might actually be a whole lot more in truth than just another great book.

Challenging Common Beliefs

The search for meaning in life is not one that is met with relative ease. Nor should it be. For those that truly desire to find their reason for being and fundamental purpose in life, the work can be arduous and requires a great deal of focus, effort, and relentless intent. It takes a call to action and a certain amount of will power that not all people on this planet possess. Unfortunately, too many people never make it to this inner calling—the deep desire to find the answer to one of the grandest questions of human existence: "Why am I here?"

For those who truly desire to understand some of the biggest questions that humans have asked themselves over the millennia, the answers can be provided. We do not need to always look to external places and other people for guidance. The answers lie within us just waiting for the proper amount of willpower and commitment from the individual seeking to understand their own truth to existence.

Like most things in life, the answers do not always come easily—at first. But with a little gentle persuasion relentlessly applied to the cause, over time, the abundance of answers can and do come flowing into the mental landscape. This is where real happiness and personal fulfillment comes from. Let us look at a few myths that need to be debunked and may even require some mental reconditioning from what we may have been brought up believing.

Myth #1—Humankind is innately bad.

This belief comes mostly from religious teachings and indoctrinations. The Bible tells of the original sin and eating the "forbidden fruit" from the "tree of knowledge of good and evil." This act cast Adam and Eve from the garden of Eden. Thus, the teachings as they have often been applied is that all humankind thereafter would also be in sin. One possible perspective to consider would be this: As mankind woke up and formed an individual consciousness, we splintered off from the Source and higher power that we are all connected to energetically. It is my belief we are still connected to that energy source, but most are oblivious to that possibility.

Our collective human consciousness decided it wanted a human experience. This does not mean we are all born sinful and innately bad people. It just means we need to live in light, love, and care to reconnect with (insert your word for God here). All human beings on Earth today have the potential to reconnect with their Source and receive direct communication and guidance in their lives. People are largely a product of their environment. What mostly makes a person evil is what has conditioned them to behave so in their individual lives. Humankind is not born evil or bad.

Myth #2—The individual is valuable.

Material things don't create the individual. We have been raised through society to believe we need to have better cars, houses, salaries, families, or even better genetics than other people in order to attain success in life. This simply is not true. The value of a person is infinite, and our true

> Money doesn't create value. The individual use of that money generates value. This can be priceless.

wealth comes from our inner potential and desire for growth and development. No amount of external riches will ever completely make a human being happy. The ability to find inner joy is what will generate real happiness and blissful peace and satisfaction in life. Jesus taught that the way to the eternal kingdom *is within you.*

Yet many of us continue to look externally. As we discussed back in chapter two, society still defines and labels people far too often by their external status. What is their title? What do they do for work? How much money do they make? These are all falsities of an individual created by the society of mankind. This is a construct, or a matrix of sorts, through which humans have defined their existence and functionality in life. None of these labels defines the value of the person. What does define us is the quality of our soul and consciousness as well as our intent at living a highly valued and morally purposeful life.

Myth #3—There are no possibilities of real positive change for the world.

Thinking that the world and the people therein cannot change is a glaring trap for overall human consciousness. That type of thinking puts people into a modality of being stuck. Humankind does not have to be doomed to suffer its own wrath. Too many people think that they are but one person—why should they try? A collective effort is essential to raise the overall human consciousness. We are all connected by energy. As one person lifts their level of vibration, it intrinsically increases the level of the conscious whole. One person is always more than zero. One hundred is better than one; one thousand is better than a hundred, and so on. We raise the overall collective consciousness on Earth by elevating the vibration one person at a time.

If we work to improve ourselves, we are making a difference on an individual and collective soul level. It may happen over longer periods of time, yet there could also be more massive jumps as group enlightenment and awakenings occur at scale. However long it will take is literally up to us—one person at a time.

Myth #4—Enlightenment is some Zenlike eternal state of consciousness.

Those seeking enlightenment have too high of an expectation due to many external impressions from different cultures. Enlightenment is not walking around every day with a massive grin on your face always in pure and everlasting contentment and heavenly euphoria. What enlightenment entails is seeking and finding your truth in life. It does involve less suffering and obtaining more happiness from a personal understanding. It is a journey that unveils new discoveries in how life is really designed along with the discoveries in truth to how the Universe works. It is within these learnings that an individual develops his or her own abilities to live masterfully in harmony with the Laws of the Universe while learning to influence these Laws to their best possible benefit.

It is quite possible that over time, the truth has been masked and hidden away from the world's population and kept secret only to those who feel they have the right to gain from these benefits. These teachings have been twisted, and a manmade spin has been placed on them by religious leaders and other similar groups. Not all of these organizations may have omitted parts of truth for their own gain. We have been made mostly to believe that fortune favors the lucky, and that we don't have much control over our lives.

We await external help and support from whatever we believe may be out there smiling down on us when in fact that power to influence and vastly shift our lives for the better lies right within our own hearts and minds. The fact of the matter is we all have an inherent right to these higher truths. It is through our personal work that we will unveil their benefits. All we need to see these truths is to start with a close look at our own belief systems and what we have been taught. We need to ask ourselves with a truly open and honest heart—have we experienced the beliefs that we have been given, or are we living through someone else's belief system hoping for good opportunities to be bestowed upon us?

I assure you this: with the right focus, willpower, and intent—you can begin to experience a positive shift in your life and career by starting your own Ungraduation and personal development process for your belief system—powered by *you*.

Ungraduated Call to Action

- Start identifying your beliefs. Make lists. You have beliefs about everything. Some support you; others don't. Select the topic areas you want to understand better (your work, your health, your relationships in general or one relationship in specific). Begin to list everything you believe about it.
- Begin to differentiate between the beliefs you list that serve you and those that limit or drain you. Notice the energetic shift when you think and write about them.
- Take any belief you hold dearly. No matter how much you might cherish the belief, ask yourself the following questions:
    1. Where did my belief come from?
    2. Is there a logical reason for holding it?
    3. Am I being limited by or elevated by this belief?
    4. What is the logical basis for holding this belief?

Chapter 11
Finding Purpose & Mission

"The two most important days in life are the day you are born and the day you find out why."
~ Mark Twain ~

It can be a sad truth that many meander through their days, weeks, months, and years without any deeper understanding of their existence. We are awarded this life to work toward meaning and purpose, yet many of us get lost as we work to find our way to "our why." There are ways of discovering our purpose that once known will yield a great deal of reward, fulfillment, and gratification within our daily lives. We are here to find that reason for being. We each have one; it is when we discover it that life takes on new meaning.

Early on in my life, I began to realize that I loved helping people. I didn't completely realize that until I got into management in the restaurant business. When I was twenty years old, I had attained the position of general manager of a restaurant. I didn't completely know how to lead at that level, but I showed up each day and gave it my best, always aiming to learn along the way. I knew that if I could attain that accomplishment at such a young age and gain some more financial freedom, I could certainly help others do it as well.

At first, it started out with me helping others attain promotions as I had done. I saw that it wasn't hard for me to move up the ranks, and with some focus and effort, I knew that others could as well. I focused on the training and development needed for interested team members. I prioritized leading others over getting promoted myself. I took great pleasure in knowing I played a role in their learning and development. My main goal was helping others, which in the long run ended up helping me just as much.

I began to forge a personal goal: I would work to help others in the fast-food world earn a good living. Ask most people if they think that one can earn a good living in fast food, and they'll either laugh or perhaps more kindly encourage a different profession for attaining life goals. I knew that in order to make a good life for myself in the world of restaurant management and leadership, I had to move up the ladder. I did just that and wanted to encourage anyone else with the heart, desire, and work ethic to do the same. It became my personal mission since I had been able to achieve it. I wanted to prove to the world that just because you work in fast food, it doesn't mean you have to be characterized as a failure.

As I worked through my career and began to achieve more and more success, it no longer was about success in the fast-food world. I wanted to make an impact in even bigger ways. I wanted to provide perspective, challenge conventional thinking, and really work with people who were seeking more meaning in life. Once one attains the basic levels of happiness and needs, what is next? That is where I now focus my attention. When people are ready, I work to help them acquire information on deeper meaning and self-exploration—to really help them find their purpose and a deeper meaning in their lives.

The Significance of the Seemingly Insignificant

We need to cherish the gift we have been given: the possibility to live with meaning. There is significance to life with all of us. The greatest sin of all may be believing we are here randomly and without purpose. We are just one species on this planet, but we interact with and change the balance of this planet through the daily decisions we put into action. Some of these decisions are more significant than others, but they all leave a lasting mark whether we realize it or not. Let us not think of our lives as insignificant. Perspective is a powerful thing. We need to take a step back to view it.

One of the shortest lifespans on planet Earth belongs to that of the mayfly. Mayflies invest a year awaiting their birth, and then within twenty-four hours, their lives end. Their sole purpose for existence is to pass on their genes. Most never even bother eating in their short lifespan. Such has been their story on Earth for nearly 100 million years.

> Knowing your "Why" is very powerful: it can be something you keep inside or share and truly become a way of life if you permit it to.

The mayfly may actually be considered one of the most evolved species on Earth when viewed through the lens of needing to pass on genes for the continuation of existence. Its sole reason for being is to ensure another generation of mayflies can see the world for another twenty-four short hours. Upon being born for one purpose—to mate—they die shortly thereafter. They have evolved to ignore the other distractions in life, such as eating, so that they can fulfill their one main objective: continuation of the species.[23]

If our lives aren't aligning with our purpose, then we can live through each day forming a means to an end. All the moments of time that pass can appear mundane as time simply passes us by. We tend to feel disconnected and weak. At the core of our lives is our purpose. When this purpose is discovered, everything in life from day-to-day waking moments to our ever-busy careers sync with that purpose so that we can act with true integrity in life. This purpose becomes our brand identity.

When we discover our purpose, then the next step is to set up the discipline so that we begin to support our most important reason for being while minimizing distractions and detractors. Once we discover our purpose or core desire in life, every moment of time we spend on it becomes a full expression of what we are seeking. When we engage in our true purpose, every moment, every instance of life is filled with the power of our hearts and determination of our minds. No longer are we simply going through the motions hoping for a means to an end. Instead, we are living the truth of our lives.

A Reason for Being—What Defines Our Purpose?

Without overthinking it, we could say that your purpose is why you get out of bed every day. It is your "Why." It is what drives you, motivates you, and compels you to be better and do better in everyday life. Once you realize this potential in yourself, you begin to understand that you can help others in that same arena. It often morphs into a service toward others. It becomes your personal brand—what you stand for and how others view you. I believe we are all living for a reason.

That reason doesn't have to be some grandiose cause for all people, though certainly it is for some. We just can't allow ourselves to get caught up in the mindset of insignificance. Many of us may never get recognized on the world stage, but make no mistake: we are all here for a curtain call. We have a purpose that placed us here, and it is up to us to find it and use that purpose for good, big or small. It all adds up in the grand scheme of life.

Aligning Your Purpose with Your Mission

The Japanese have a term for how to find one's reason for being. They term this purpose *Ikigai*. At its core, *Ikigai* is a lifestyle practice through which we find balance in our career and personal passions. When we are in balance with the flow of our purpose, we are monetized and rewarded for helping solve a need in the world. The history of the practice of *Ikigai* dates to the Heian period (794 to 1185 present era). The word *Gai* in Japanese comes from the word *Kai* (meaning shell). During this era in Japanese history, shells were deemed valuable and used as a currency. The word *Ikigai* derived from this terminology and into a word meaning "value in living."[24]

The history of *Ikigai* has taken on new meaning over the last few decades as it has been westernized and taught by human resource managers, life coaches, and many self-help teachers to generate a better work–life balance. This life philosophy is one that can and does help many figure out why they get out of bed each morning.

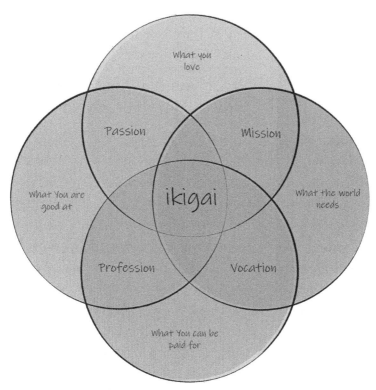

The current model of *Ikigai* has four components:
- What are you doing that you love?
- Are you doing what the world needs?
- What are you doing that you are good at?
- What are you doing that you can be paid for?

In its original intent, *Ikigai* was not needing to have all four components active for one to achieve purpose. However, this modernized, westernized version paints a beautiful picture for what we would strive to attain in life. It is a great depiction of what trying to attain balance in life looks like.

It is quite OK to not have all of these elements in perfect balance. The diagram above depicts what we all should strive for but isn't 100% necessary for happiness. If you aren't in a profession that you feel is aligned to your life purpose, use your skills and natural gifts to make the most amount of impact within that profession. I can speak to this from personal experience.

In my more than twenty years of working in the restaurant business, I was largely responsible for driving sales, operations, and profitability in the restaurants I was responsible for. While this was the overarching objective I had to deliver on, I realized that I could achieve this goal through focusing on helping people with their personal development. The teachings and perspective I gave them in turn not only helped them run better operations but also helped them to think differently. It would challenge their conventional thoughts, and that gave them the opportunity to grow and learn. That became the driving force for what I would do each day at work. I didn't set out to drive sales and profit—I set out to drive personal development and leadership. That in turn improved their business, which of course helped the company achieve its goals.

> When you find your North Star, it will burn so brightly in your life that you'll never be lost.

Regardless of how you view the concept, it is a powerful and beneficial way to frame your views on life, purpose, and mission. After all, it is really about what motivates you when you wake up every morning. It is essential to realize that we need not get caught up in this grandiose expectation that everything must perfectly align and stay in balance. Is this possible? Absolutely, but we need not set ourselves up for expectations that may lead to frustrations and then dismissal of the basic principles. The key is to investigate specific areas of our life to help define what it is that we are seeking to accomplish.

Framing Your Purpose & Mission

I like to think of three main areas of focus when we are aiming to discover our life purpose and mission. These three buckets are what we can use to help us frame up our purpose, *Ikigai*, or reason for being. It correlates purposefully to W.H.Y.—our reason for being:

- **W**orld needs this.
- **H**eed your talents.
- **Y**earn after your passions in life

What Are the Needs of the World?

We begin with pondering on how we can make the world a better place. Again, we don't need to focus too large at this point. All we need to do is take a step back and think about issues in the world that we would like to see improve. There will likely be many, but we begin with creating a list of items that we feel can be better. We may look at certain aspects of life and just say, "Why can't *xyz* be better?" Think of it in terms of how inventors disrupt the business world. The smartphone started out as a phone but evolved into a personal device that disrupted countless other categories in the business world. Had someone not thought of the internet, perhaps the smartphone wouldn't have been created. Maybe we'd still be sending handwritten letters back and forth rather than instant email messages.

The point here is obvious: we want to think of ways we can improve the way of doing things. Ideas then can be built upon each other and soon morph into completely new aspects of everyday life. Make a list of the aspects of life in the world that you feel can and should be better. Don't limit yourself. Write out all that comes into your stream of consciousness.

Heeding Your Talents

Now it is time to list what you are really good at. This can be a difficult step for some because most of us are naturally wired to see what we aren't good at first. This is a step through which we have to really celebrate ourselves a bit. Each of us is talented in some aspect of our lives.

If you are really struggling here, ask yourself what others often thank you for. What do they stop and give you accolades for? At work, what do your colleagues point out that you do very well? Perhaps your friends recognize these traits in you and have told you in the past how they appreciate aspects of your character.

We all have talents that provide a service to others. This is the time to celebrate yourself a little. Quite frankly, we don't make enough time in our lives for this. Now is as good a time as ever to take a few moments and jot down what it is that you really know you are good at.

If you get stuck, you might want to use some of the great tools online. One I have used in the past is Strengthsfinder 2.0 from Tom Rath. Tom has a book on the subject of discovering your strengths that I always recommend as a way to discover how to begin leveraging your strengths to your advantage. There is even a free assessment you can take at https://high5test.com/strengthsfinder-free/. The key in this step is to begin to pay attention, take notice of, and heed our talents to our advantage and to benefit the lives of others.

Yearning After Your Passions in Life

Once we understand what the world needs and what talents we can provide to the world, it is time to apply those two elements to your passion or calling in life. This is where we look at the aspects of our lives around which we have strong desires and feelings. What do you have an intense yearning or longing for in life?

For example, I am deeply passionate about trying to find answers to some of the biggest questions to humankind's existence.

- Who and what are we, really?
- Why are we here?
- Who or what brought us to this place?
- What happens once our physical existence on this Earth is no more?

I know these are deep questions about life, but they are my passion and part of my yearning for purpose and reason for being. Along with seeking these answers for myself, I aim to bring others along for the ride.

We don't need to have big, overarching passions. Our passions can be around being the best mother or father possible to our children. Maybe becoming the best software designer is something that drives the inner purpose of a computer programmer. Perhaps you are passionate about sustainability and how we can better leave our planet to the next generation. It could really be as simple as being passionate about learning one new thing today that you didn't know yesterday.

The best part about defining your passions is that *they are yours*. It doesn't matter what others think of them or how they perceive your passions. This is where you get to define your life purpose on your terms. Allow no one to influence you in this regard. You can share your passions and talk about them with others; just know they may be quick to give thoughts and feedback. Don't let their reactions sway you in your determination for what brings you excitement.

Forming Your Purpose & Mission Statement

Once you have completed a list of world needs, heeded talents you possess, and taken notice of where you yearn for certain passions in life to be pursued, it is time to form a purpose and mission statement. We want to begin with looking at each of the three categories and start to form a statement from them. Some like to form separate purpose and mission statements. Certainly, you could form your purpose statement and then the mission behind it. To me, they are one and the same. This is your purpose and mission in life and no one else's. Make this about you and what works for you only. Below is an example of my current purpose and mission statement:

> Inspire others to seek out new learning perspectives that challenge limiting life beliefs—in order to discover new and empowering personal awakenings that lead them to complete happiness, prosperity, and fulfillment of their life purpose.

Here is how this purpose statement was formed:

- World need—Individual personal awakenings toward happiness, prosperity, and life purposes.
- Heeding my talent—Inspirational learning and teaching of new life perspectives.
- Yearning after passion in life—eliminating the limiting, preprogrammed societal life beliefs we have.

You get to have fun with this creative process and insert the action words that form the complete purpose & mission statement. Try not to overthink it. Enjoy the process. Your purpose and mission statement will evolve and change over time. That is perfectly normal. Since I began this process of working to live with more meaning in my life, my own purpose statement has had about a dozen different iterations.

Once you get comfortable with a purpose and mission statement that seems to incorporate your list of world needs, heeded talents, and your yearning passions, print that bad boy, and get it up somewhere you will see it every day.

I printed mine on a small baseball-card-sized printout and was able to slide it into a plastic holder that I could carry in my shirt pocket.

You just want to get used to seeing your reason for being in a place that will remind you of what you have committed to make more of a difference in life.

Once you do this, you will be reminded daily and begin to see your life take shape with more meaning and purpose. If you live with this purpose in mind each day and truly exemplify it in as many ways as possible, you will begin to feel and understand your *real meaning*. The rewards will come back to you as you provide a service to others. You will begin to witness the Principle of Correspondence in action as you will receive abundance for your actions. You will begin to work in true balance with the Universe.

> Pay attention to the impulses that pop up around you; these could be signs from the universe to take action on new beneficial opportunities.

This is a huge step for you. If you get to this point of perspective in your life, congratulations. You are one of the few—part of the few that I am hoping to see become many more. You will begin to feel what true happiness, success, and purpose are like. Be proud of your accomplishment. Wear that badge of achievement with pride. You are now one of the few who has discovered their purpose and mission in life.

Ungraduated Call to Action

It's time to figure out your "Why" and write your purpose statement:

- What does the world need?

  Think about the aspects of life you would like to improve for yourself, loved ones, business, or circle of influence. Write these ideas down. Don't limit yourself. Dream big here. It doesn't have to impact the world on a global scale but needs to be something that you jump out of bed for each day excited to take on.

- Heed your talents.

  Be it through the Strengthsfinder assessment or your own perspective, what talents do you have that can lend you advantages along your journey toward solving your world need? Ask others in your close circle what it is that they think are some of your skills and talents in life. List them out.

- What passions do you yearn after in life?

  Now jot down some aspects you are passionate about related to solving your world need. These are the things that drive that "fire in the belly." When the going gets tough, as it inevitably will, these passions are what will fuel you in your fight to solve your world need.

- From your list of world needs, talents, and passions, let's take some of each and formulate a few sentences. Try to keep it to three or four sentences. First, what passions do you have along with talents to impact and improve upon your world need?

Don't worry about being perfect in this process. Once you have something down on paper, post it or print it so you can keep it with you or have it somewhere you'll see each day. As you work toward your goals, this can certainly be tweaked and improved.

Chapter 12

Living an Ungraduated Mindset Daily

"It is entirely possible that behind the perception of our senses, worlds are hidden of which we are unaware."
~ Albert Einstein ~

If you have made it this far, congratulations! You are on your way to a new unconventional, Ungraduated way to put the control of your life back where it always belonged—not in your hands, but in your head as your new personal belief system. You now know that as you think it, you become it.

There are a great many distractions on this journey we call life that will aim to pull you back off course. Life in the twenty-first century is designed in such a way that we quickly become distracted. However, we can successfully navigate the waters. We can recognize and avoid the temptations that pull our powerful intentions away from control of our own life and toward the mental constructs of others. Those mental constructs will quickly shackle us back into the realm of the lost and disillusioned.

Living an Ungraduated life becomes a natural daily occurrence when we keep our awareness pointed toward the direction of self-empowerment. Even when challenges or the distractions in life are placed in front of us, with the proper mental framing, we will always stay in control. Living with an Ungraduated mindset means paying attention to what life places in front of us. We need to now become the watchers of the shadows of life, carefully observing what is creeping from behind us and then into our peripheral field of vision. When we cast our thoughts and desires out into the Universe, we then need to become observant of how answers and opportunities will be placed into our everyday lives.

Surrendering to the Flow of Life

One of my all-time favorite books, *The Surrender Experiment* by Michael Singer, frames this perspective perfectly. In this amazing real-life story, Michael speaks to his observation of life and how taking the necessary leaps of faith led him from one life accomplishment to the next. He set sail on the winds of faith. Those winds carried him across the ocean of possibilities, stopping for new discoveries and learnings along the way. In his book, Michael describes mostly being focused on meditation and trying to connect with his higher purpose. All he is interested in is helping others discover the peace and serenity that he has discovered through his practices. He sets out to grow his meditation practice, and one opportunity after the next helps him achieve his goals of growing his following and teachings. Soon, he is building larger buildings through his skill of carpentry and helping others explore the many benefits of meditation along with him.

It wasn't until after he *surrendered* to the flow of life that he began receiving answers and gifts at almost every turn and in the most serendipitous ways. One might assume these open pathways might be many strokes of luck and coincidence—that is, as I stated earlier in my own experiences in life, until the number of coincidences become mathematically improbable.

At one point in his life, Michael walked past a storefront window and saw a display set up containing a twelve-inch screen hooked up to a TRS-80 computer. Not even really understanding what a computer was, he felt the strange nudge from his gut instinct to purchase it, assuming he'd have a need for it at some point down the road. He became fascinated with the possibilities it yielded, so

Michael set off to generate a new software program that would help him keep track of his carpentry business. Word began to travel, and he received numerous requests from medical practices for a similar program that would help them keep track of their medical billing and record keeping. Before his very eyes, the Universe continued handing Michael one amazing opportunity after another.

Eventually, Michael found himself in a prestigious, high-level executive position and running his own independent publicly traded software company. Later in his book, he tells more of his story from here and how it took an unexpected turn for the worse with a lawsuit and potential jail time due to one of his employees involved in fraud and bribery. Even with this challenge, easily viewed negatively by most, Michael was given the next opportunity as he was forced to step aside as CEO from his multimillion-dollar business.

Because the lawsuits took years to unfold, he was able to use his newfound spare time to write *The Untethered Soul*, a book that became a *New York Times* best seller. This book took him on his next purpose, as he was able to continue to help others transform their lives through his story and teaching with a much larger following and platform.

The key takeaway from Michael and his two *New York Times* bestselling books *The Untethered Soul* and *The Surrender Experiment*, is this: allow life to flow. Pay attention to what life is placing in front of you. Situations and coincidences have more meaning than we may perhaps realize. Say *yes* to life more than *no*, and watch in amazement as opportunities unfold before your eyes.

The Four Quadrants of Ungraduated Living

When put into place, four main aspects of daily practice will ensure that we stay in an aware state of mind and in control of our life manifestations. Through putting attention, practice, and effort behind these four daily aspects, we can ensure that we keep control of our lives and our purpose behind living.

Mindset

How we perceive our world determines how we interact with it. Ever wake up to a gloomy, overcast, rainy day? Sure, we all have—unless perhaps you live in a desert without even the occasional monsoon. Assuming you aren't living among the cacti of the hot and dry desert plains, most often we see a rainy, gloomy day as depressing and undesirable.

The key for us to begin bringing more positivity into our lives is to rewire our perceived negative aspects of life. The rain is nourishing and peaceful rather than undesirable and a nuisance. The traffic you are sitting in as you commute home from work is an opportunity to take a moment of pause and reflection. Perhaps listen to an audiobook or download your favorite podcast rather than slamming your fists into the dashboard.

How we frame our mindset in the present moment is what dictates our outcomes. We control our choices and our perceptions of the world we see each day. What lies outside of our control is simply a choice for us in how we perceive it. That rainy day—just another opportunity to see the front yard becoming greener and your plants and flowers growing with its nourishment. The traffic you are stuck in right now—only a chance to relax and listen to your favorite song on your music playlist.

Heartset

As we discussed in chapter seven, we can align our hearts to our minds for maximum synchronization. When we live through feeling our purpose from our heart, we are guided each day toward more potentiality.

I can personally speak to this aspect in my own present moment. I've known for years that I wanted to help make a difference for others beyond just the day job I have leading others in the restaurant business. I just didn't know what avenue I needed to go down in order to expand beyond my current level of impact.

Through the self-synchronization techniques taught in chapter seven, I have been able to align my mindset with my heartset. As we open to these possibilities, we find ourselves reading the books we need, listening to the helpful podcasts, finding the right mastermind group to join, signing up for the best seminars, meeting the people who present us the proper relationships we need to help us attain our purpose. This is the magic of aligning our hearts with our minds. We aren't just driven by random spontaneous thought, or by misguided emotional feelings from the heart. When the heart and mind are in line and communicating, we are led to more fulfillment and discovery.

This is precisely what has led me to this point in my own life. My heart is now leading me along the path I need to walk in order to attain more of my life purpose. It started with getting my mindset right more than ten years ago, and then as I learned to synchronize my heart to my mind in the daily practice described in chapter seven, I then began to be led to the discoveries I needed in order to achieve more purpose.

When I got serious about paying attention to what life was putting in front of me through my mindset and meditating on those decisions through the connection to my heartset, I began to hear the Universe speaking to me. I describe this as a deep knowing of a certain answer or level of guidance. Knowing it when you *feel it* is the only way I can describe it. Here is a real-life example of how this worked in my life.

Before I came to the realization that I was going to write a book, I only had the perspective from my mindset that I wanted to help people. I thought about how to help people I worked with and led. That was my motivation for a long time. But I still felt a hollowness inside—even with the good I was doing with the people I mentored at work.

So, I began to meditate daily on my heart–mind connection. I put the thoughts from my mind into my heart. I deeply put out the message to the Universe in five-to-ten-minute meditations that I needed to find more meaning and influence. I knew there was more of a purpose for me than my current responsibilities and desperately wanted to be led to it.

Without knowing exactly why, I developed in interest in cryptocurrency. A friend I worked with turned me on to it during the first big run up with bitcoin in late 2017, so I decided to invest some money into it. Due to the high volatility and risk involved, I didn't put in more than I was comfortable with losing.

I watched in amusement as my investment rode the choppy waves of the blockchain world. It rose and fell, rose some more, and then fell in a big way. I let that investment sit, determined that it would pay off. Something in me told me it would.

Through that experience, I came across Overstock and learned about how the online retail chain had been licking its wounds from the massive online retail giant war mostly won by Amazon. Overstock had decided to form a branch of its business ventures in the crypto space and align with becoming more of a blockchain-based business. The stock price had already plummeted from its all-time high of around $85 a share to trading around $20 a share. Something told me to invest and buy some stock. Again, I invested a relatively small amount in the company and acquired about one hundred shares. I watched with more amusement as the stock price fell to $15 and eventually $10. I even bought some more stock when it hit $9, assuming it couldn't go much lower. Then it sank to around $3.

I had pretty much assumed my adventures in trading and listening to my heart had been a massive mistake. Since I had already ridden these investments so low, I decided to continue to just bleed out my total investment to zero if necessary. Perhaps it was my stubbornness, but again, something told me, "Just hang in there. It's all going to work out soon."

By that time, the COVID-19 pandemic had fully enmeshed itself into our everyday lives. Everyone was working from home and ordering online. The sudden realization that life would go on—just differently—had been realized. People flooded the internet as they aimed to complete all those home projects they had been putting off for a rainy day. Overstock.com shot through the roof and hit new all-time highs of around $125 a share. The panic of the sudden global economic uncertainty had propelled bitcoin to new all-time highs as well. Suddenly the price of one bitcoin was going for around $66k. That was a far cry from the initial purchase price when I had taken a relatively small investment and placed the purchase of two bitcoin.

Now, I didn't turn into a master online trader of company stock and bitcoin overnight. I didn't buy at the lowest price and sell at the highest. That part of the investment payout was far from perfect, but I did end up making enough money to put to good use. I joined a few mastermind groups that surrounded me with people that can help me with my entrepreneurial goals. Through these connections, I am learning to create websites, generate and host a podcast, as well as many other aspects that are helping me fulfill the purpose of spreading my Ungraduated Living & Learning message to others.

Coincidence, you might say, but I think not. The first mastermind I joined was the first I had ever heard of. It also required a significant investment to be a part of it with an annual membership. Even though my wife and I are blessed with enough funds to have purchased that mastermind membership, it wouldn't have happened without those investments paying off. We have too many other financial goals such as paying off our home mortgage. Those priorities take center stage right now over all else. So, I knew if I approached her about wanting to invest some of our savings to join a mastermind—it would have been a big no from her. And nothing against the love of my life; she would have been right, as we both agreed to commit to the paying off of our home so we can be 100% debt free.

The first mastermind I joined propelled me to learn and grow in ways that have enabled me to begin the next phase of my life purpose and potential. I am meeting and connecting with the exact people I need to help me accomplish my current goals. Many people would look at the significant price tag of a meeting group and call me crazy. However, there is no price not worth paying if it means attaining the life of complete meaning, fulfillment, happiness, and purpose that I aim to achieve.

When you are in complete alignment from your heartset to your mindset, life will align for you in the ways it needs to. Money will come when you most need it. Connections will unfold in front of you that lead to the right people. Opportunities will present themselves and take you to where you need to be. All you have to do is pay attention.

Perhaps *paying attention* is actually the highest price tag of all.

So very few of us in life stop to recognize the journey life is telling us to take. Who knows the cost that mounts from lost opportunities and wasted life purpose—for me, I'm sure it will be worth a lot more than the investment of a mastermind.

Healthset

The well-known phrase of, "You can't take care of anyone else before you take care of yourself" rings very true. These physical vessels we call our bodies have been afforded to us during our physical adventure of life. We need to care for our bodies at a basic and essential level. Failure to recognize this not only can lend itself to our failure in achieving our life purpose, but also personal challenges that will take us off course, or worse, an early termination of our time on earth.

We need to ensure we do the best we can with proper nutrition, physical activity, and sleep. When we are aligned with the right mindset and heartset, we can begin to pay attention to what our physical bodies need. What we want to accomplish is working more toward taking the daily vitamin rather than needing the pain pill later in life.

I can again tie this back to my own journey in life as we visited earlier. As I started to align my heartset and mindset a few years ago, I began to have a very strong desire to get myself in better shape. For years I had been wanting to eat better, get better sleep, and exercise more regularly. I just had not made the commitment. There were always excuses—too much travel, too many late-night business dinners I had to attend, too much work in any given day to make more time for my body and health.

Working on your body will become a part of your life once you are aligned in your mindset and heartset. You won't be able to do one without the other. You wouldn't want to walk out of a gym and light up a smoke, much as you will find yourself gravitating toward better care of your physical health once you get your mindset and heartset in order.

This is how it happened for me. It was December 26, 2019, when I stepped off the weighing platform of truth called a bathroom scale and decided I needed to make changes for my physical health. The connection of my mind to my heart called into action the need to better my physical body. Besides, the scale got tired of hearing me asking it why it was always lying to me. I accepted that at 6' 0" and 250 pounds, I was overweight. The scale had been telling me the truth after all.

In my short moments of meditation, I began receiving the necessary information of what my body needed to get healthy. Insights came to me that seemed difficult to make changes around, but I knew I was receiving the guidance I needed. I discovered David Asprey's book, *Super Human*. Within that book are so many tips to help slow the aging process and give your body the nutrients it needs for ultimate health and wellness. Dave Asprey confidently describes his goal to live to the age of 160. With the right mindset and determination, I believe the goal of living vibrantly beyond the age of 100 or even 120 is very doable.

We have to remember, we program our bodies through our minds. Society has us believing that certain age groups are old. What defines "old"? Well, of course, for starters, the average lifespan of a human is where we start. But why must we adhere to old beliefs that we can't live with good mind, body, and soul into our 100s and beyond? Remember the Principle of Polarity we discussed from chapter three; numbers are often relative. When does "old" become "old?" We base labels concerning age off predetermined perspectives of our recorded history. At one point in human history, you were perceived old if you made it to fifty.

It does take physical action to accomplish goals like David's, but with the right alignment of mindset and heartset, I believe we can begin to slow the aging process and then redefine what age group we fall into. This type of Ungraduated thinking and living is how we lend ourselves to begin looking like we are twenty years old at thirty, then thirty years old at forty. At one point, the age of one hundred may appear to be only seventy or eighty.

We don't need to fall into the mental constructs of what we've been told to believe. With the right alignment of mental focus and physical action, we can rewrite the expectations on aging. With this newfound information well entrenched into my mindset and heartset, I set out to make changes to my healthset. I have touched on some of these changes in a previous chapter, but for the sake of complete understanding, I'll share more depth to the story.

First, I decided right then and there I was going to cut back on my alcohol intake. I was using my social drinking as a crutch for destressing myself after a long week. No longer would I have to drink on the weekends in order to wind down from the week. Besides, those weekend winddowns had turned into almost daily winddowns.

Enough was enough.

Along with the decision to cut back on drinking came the decision to stop drinking soda. No matter the type, regular or diet, I was done with it. Cold turkey, hard stop. From that day on, I would drink mostly water throughout the day. I ordered a home water filter for filtration of my tap water and began getting reacquainted with our good friend H_2O.

In addition, I had the insight that I should cut out all deep-fried foods. This one was more difficult than deciding to stop drinking soda and limiting alcohol. But I made the decision, my wife purchased us an air fryer, and away I went on the pursuit of this goal. I have been nearly perfect since that decision, but not 100%. There are rare occasions when I'm out for dinner and indulge in one or two truffle oil French fries. But I am 99% in the camp of no longer eating deep-fried food.

Then came the most difficult decision. I would no longer consume any mammal meat of any kind. I still eat fish, but no mammals. This was more of a moral decision for me than that of a health decision. Without going too much into the story here, I decided I could no longer be a hypocrite who loves animals and yet consume them for breakfast, lunch, and dinner.

Lastly, I made the commitment to begin every day with a minimum of forty-five minutes of some type of physical activity. No matter what I had planned for the day, I would wake up as early as necessary to complete at least forty-five minutes of stationary bike riding, jogging, elliptical, etc. Through to the day of this writing, I have not missed a day and do not intend to. That's right—no days off.

What resulted over the following weeks and months was astounding. Without fail, I would lose 2 pounds a week or roughly 8–10 pounds a month. From January 2020 through the end of June 2020, I was down 60 pounds. The transformation was invigorating. I felt clearer of mind and could focus more intently on tasks at hand. I had more physical energy. I began to love my body, perhaps for the first time in my life.

All those around me noticed the changes, too. Like most who achieve a rapid and noticeable physical transformation, I was being asked what I had done differently. Over the now hundreds of times I've been asked, I simply repeated the aforementioned changes.

When I would rattle off a few of the first decisions, heads would nod. But as I got through the list, most head nods would shift to head shakes—with comments like, "Wow, not sure I can commit to that." I assured all those then and those reading now, you most absolutely can do these things and more if you desire it. It simply comes down to how aware you are of your purpose on this planet. If one is not aligned within their mindset and heartset, then it may become likely that they don't commit to the necessary physical changes for the betterment of their body and health. However, once that first step is taken, it becomes impossible *not to make the necessary life changes for the betterment of your health and body.*

While these health changes don't occur overnight, we must remember that through thought, our daily actions make up our futures. If you want to make change in your future, you do so through everyday decisions. It simply comes down to how badly you want it—or better put—how aligned you are within your mindset and heartset.

Soulset

Robin Sharma once said, "A bad day for the ego is a great day for the soul." This is the focus of the fourth and final category of living an Ungraduated life. Once we can balance our mindset, heartset, and healthset, it is time to turn our attention very much inward—toward our soul or spirit.

One of the most life-changing books I ever read is Eckhart Tolle's *Power of Now*. As if teaching that the present moment and removing ourselves from thoughts in the past and toward the present isn't profound enough, Eckhart also reveals the biggest enemy each of us have hiding away inside our heads: the ego. The "inner chatter" that we all have, the voice inside our heads.

The goal of aligning to our soulset is to quiet the inner voice and constant self-talk from which the ego thrives. Don't misconstrue the ego as the voice that is always clambering for more attention, the voice that overpowers the human being and is always needing the limelight. That is one form of how the ego expresses itself, but there are many others. The ego is also responsible for keeping us entrenched in mediocrity. It is the voice that tells us we aren't good enough to try new things. We'll likely fail and look silly if we step outside of our comfort zone. It is the voice of temptation to go against your moral values, telling you, "You will never know unless you try." Since discovering and really analyzing the ego, I have often wondered if the ego is the biblical description of the devil. The parallels of similarity are uncanny.

Making time to develop a practice of meditation and prayer is key to the development of your soulset. I contrast prayer and meditation as prayer is the act of you asking for guidance from (insert your word for God here), while meditation is the practice through which you receive your answers. Meditation need not be difficult or hard. It is our ego that gets in the way and prevents us from casting the bright light into its corner. For the ego understands quite well once that light is shining, its power and control is lessened.

Ego identifies itself through the five senses of the physical world: sight, sound, taste, touch, and smell. Your soulset identifies itself through the connection beyond the physical world. Much of humanity still mainly exists mentally within the constructs of the physical world only. Through the Principle of Cause and Effect, we begin to understand that when we put attention on that of the nonphysical mental planes, we will start to experience the result of that focus from the mental plane back to the physical realms.

When we dedicate small amounts of time to the practice of prayer or meditation, we begin to quiet the ego. We can become more in tune with our higher selves and that of our calling and purpose. The ego is pushed aside.

> It is what it is—when you live life with acceptance of "what is," that is the end of all drama in your life.

It may never cease to exist, but your guiding light builds through that of the soul and your purpose, rather than that of confusion from the ego. You will feel more "called upon." You will see more of the avenues you must travel down. More bridges of opportunity will open up for you. The elements of your life will take on more synchronicity to bring you what you need for your own growth, development, and opportunities.

This is how we accomplish living with a daily Ungraduated mindset. The noise and chatter of external distractions begin to slowly quiet and fade away. We then begin to see and hear with more clarity than ever as our paths become illuminated with clarity and understanding. No longer do we feel we are meandering about aimlessly. We see the distractions of the manmade world for what they are, speedbumps built into the highway of our lives only meant to slow us down. We now feel enlightened and emboldened to live life on our terms. The speedbumps are removed from our life highways and the speed limit signs along with them. We are free to travel toward our goals, full of clear meaning and purposeful intent.

Epilogue & Ungraduation

"The real voyage of discovery consists not in seeking new lands but in seeing with new eyes."
~ Marcel Proust ~

I want to thank you for making it this far with me. It is my hope that this book has presented a challenging, new way of approaching everyday life, a new way of perceiving what the world places in front of you. The world itself is up for interpretation—your interpretation. Not the interpretation of what others in the world want or expect you to believe. You are formatting your own outcomes. Others in this world will often try to formulate your opinions and place you back into a limiting life belief system, but you will now see that for the trap it is. You are now viewing the world through a new and empowering light. You have the ability to create and manifest your boundless potential and purpose in life.

Going all the way on your journey requires knowing your "Why." It is the reason for your being, the purpose for why you begin to walk your path in the first place. It is my hope that this book has helped provide some answers.

> *Veri veniversum virus vici:*
> **By the power of truth, I, while living, have conquered the universe.**

However, if it has fulfilled its true purpose, you now have more questions. That is the very point of this book.

While I have aimed to try to frame up how life has worked for me, I very much want to generate thought and motivating questions for you to seek answers to. What has worked for me will likely work for others, but we are all walking our own journeys of self-discovery.

Not every person is going to be the same in what they need for their own Ungraduation and personal awakening in life. I sincerely hope that I have driven you to the starting point of your own personal Ungraduation from the old system of thought and indoctrination.

There are only two mistakes on the path to truth: not starting down the path and not completing the journey.

I hope you have enjoyed this self-discovery and true awakening of new perspectives on life. It is my wish and desire that you continue to question more in your life, seek out new perspectives, and formulate your own truths. Becoming Ungraduated in your life and learning is a lifelong process. You have taken the first steps and have begun the journey to personal truth. Where will you go from here? The choice, as in all things in life, is up to you.

> The awakened person is the greatest stranger in the world. They do not seem to belong to anybody—no organization, community, society, or nation confines them.
> —Osho

Acknowledgments

It is said that around 80% of people want to write a book. Yet only a small fraction of that population does.

It is my belief that a thought is the beginning of a waveform of potentiality. It is when these thoughts fester, resonate, and are dwelled upon that they become more powerful. If strong enough and believed in enough, these thoughts then turn into life purposes, through which we bring action into the equation. These actions are what begin cementing the possible outcomes of potentiality into one finite outcome. A thought is simply that—a thought. Through taking action, waveforms of thoughts and potentialities then become matter, or simply put, part of the physical world. This is the result of manifesting our thoughts, hopes, and dreams into our realities.

The reality of this book would not be possible without the following very important and special higher-self connections and individuals in my life.

First, my own personal awakening, the connectedness to the calling that I felt from my higher self, my Source, the Universe, the divine, God. Since the first thought entered my head some 15+ years ago that there is far more going on in the world than meets the physical eye, I have searched for and been led to more truths and discoveries through this connection with my higher self. This connection to a higher power has been guiding my life for some time now and has serendipitously positioned me to meet the right people and the proper time in my life to bring this book into reality. For the discovery of this connection to all things infinite, I will be forever grateful.

A big part of my own personal awakening has been the most important person in my life. My love, my reason for being, my everything, my loving life partner in life: Crystal. You came into my life just as I was starting to think as an adult. I was determined ever so much to make it in what we call this human experience called life along your side. You supported me along the way and trusted in me whenever I gave you many reasons to doubt me. Thank you for having faith in me, supporting me, guiding me, and being such an amazing best friend and wife. There is no greater gift in life than having a love who is also your best friend and partner for life.

To my family: my mother Nancy, father Joel, stepfather Bob, stepmother Ellen, mother-in-law Martha-Jean, and father-in-law Joe. Whether realized or not, each of you have played an integral role in shaping me into the person I've become today. The many different life experiences along our paths have not all been easy, yet I would never change any single outcome. It is through you all that my life lived has defined my personal character and the individual I've become. Thank you all for doing your absolute best to provide me perspective, love, understanding, and guidance. A special thanks to Martha-Jean and Joe. Without each of you, I would not have the love of my life, Crystal. Thank you both not only for her but also for being such amazing in-laws.

To my brother Tim: I am grateful for our conversations about life and higher-level perspectives. Whether you realize it or not, you have helped me to see my own struggles around ego and the need to resist its urges to persuade others that I am right and they are wrong. I know we don't see everything in alignment with each other's views, but that is perfect in and of itself and how we all grow in learning and understanding. It is through staying open-minded toward other people's perspectives that helps us grow, and you have played a role in my growth, development, and spiritual awakening through our conversations.

A very special thank you to Kent Sanders of the Daily Writer Community. It was through you and your unending belief that everyone should indeed write a book that I began to see the potential in myself to write a book as well. Here again, serendipity played a massive role. It was through my good friend and mentor Tommy Breedlove that I met you. You helped me see this task in small bite-sized steps that helped me frame up the perspective I needed to bring this book into life. This is the first book in my life, and certainly not going to be my last thanks to my learnings from you and your Daily Writer Community.

For my friend and mentor Tommy Breedlove: thank you for helping me see myself as "Legendary." All of humanity has the potential to become Legendary, but you help the select few that truly want it to decide, commit, and succeed in legendary ways. I've become better as a person and leader from meeting you. I appreciate our friendship and our Legendary Community and am grateful for your continued love, support, and encouragement for me throughout this process.

I am fortunate to have not only one great mentor in life, but two. I'm thankful for having met my second mentor in my life, Vincent Pugliese. Vincent and his "Total Life Freedom" community again found me, rather than me finding them. I believe Vincent and his community came into my life just when I needed it most. It is through Vincent and his community that I am aiming to bring my messages and teachings into life in entrepreneurial ways, that I hope can help reach more people needing it. Thank you, Vincent, to you and your community members who are helping me realize my fullest potential, to not only venture into entrepreneurship, but so many other valuable aspects of life, leadership, and learning.

Any good book needs a good editor, and for me, that was Jennifer Harshman and her team at Harshman Services. I could not have found a better editor for my needs. You took my ball of clay and helped me finish it into the product that is being held in the hands of the reader this very moment. You are all truly exceptional at what you do, and I am excited for future opportunities to work with you. You are some of the best in the business! Thank you!

Last, but far from being least, is my corporate team I work alongside in the restaurant business. There are far too many names to put here for the acknowledgments, for it would probably take up half the book. But each one of you knows who you are. Thank you for giving me the grace and understanding, and for humoring me in our many philosophical conversations and points of view. I appreciate the opportunity to lead and work alongside you all and intend to continue to be the best leader, peer, and friend for you until the Universe decides it is no longer necessary. Even when and if that day comes, I'll be honored to still call you all friends for life.

About the Author

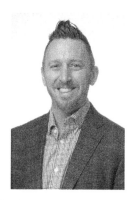

Ken Hannaman is an executive leader in the restaurant industry with the responsibility of 700+ restaurants. In addition to his corporate responsibilities, he is also an author, writer, and possibility mindset coach.

He is the husband to his wife and life partner Crystal, having enjoyed life together for 24+ years. Neither of them has navigated life on traditional terms. Ken dropped out of high school and upon meeting Crystal, became aware that she never wanted to have children. Together, they have marched against social norms and have forged a life well lived on their own terms, defined through them, and away from societal labels.

Ken has a real-life "nothing to everything" story. It has been through his relationships in the many different levels he's held in his corporate career that he's had the ability to reflect on what in life has made him successful. Having met, coached, and observed the lives and careers of thousands of different individuals, Ken has come to the realization that happiness, purpose, health and wellness, along with personal and professional success are all the result of mindset and belief systems.

We often allow our lives to be defined by others, through education, religion, governments, and other organizations that indoctrinate us into the belief that life is best lived one way—their way. Ken helps others find their way through their "Why."

It just requires a little bit of Ungraduation from the old views of a bygone era and the ability to see with new eyes how we shape our lives for the better or for the worse through our belief systems.

Through his own life experiences and rewiring of his own programming, Ken has broken free of the outdated belief systems that were holding him back from all his life passions and desires. This, his first book, is a result of his own inner work, reflection, and real-life learnings that he hopes will inspire others to discover that the lives they so desire are not in their hands, but rather mostly in their heads.

Endnotes

Chapter 1

1 file: ///Volumes/Lexar/Ungraduated% 20Book/Book% 20Reference% 20Links/Michelson-Morley% 20experiment/ Case% 20Western% 20Reserve% 20University% 20-% 20Michelson-Morley% 20experiment.html
https: //www.thoughtco.com/the-michelson-morley-experiment-2699379

2 file: ///Volumes/Lexar/Ungraduated% 20Book/Book% 20Reference% 20Links/Higgs% 20boson% 20field/The% 20Higgs% 20boson% 20_% 20CERN.html
https: //www.science20. com/alpha_meme/higgs_discovery_rehabilitating_despised_einstein_ether-85497
https: //home.cern/news/series/lhc-physics-ten/higgs-boson-what-makes-it-special

3 https://www.wired.com/2014/12/fantastically-wrong-thing-evolution-darwin-really-screwed/

4 https://www.americanrhetoric.com/speeches/teddyrooseveltmuckrake.htm

5 https://books.google.com/books? id=Arsc2H9_KwC&newbks=0&hl=en&source=newbks_fb

Chapter 2

6 https://www.simplypsychology.org/milgram.html

7 https://www.history.com/topics/religion/zoroastrianism

8 History.com Editors. "Zoroastrianism." History.com. A&E Television Networks, February 13, 2018. https://www.history.com/topics/religion/zoroastrianism.

9 https://www.thoughtco.com/great-compromise-of-1787-3322289

Chapter 3

10 https://www.delawarepublic.org/post/why-doesnt-your-butt-fall-through-chair

11 https://choosemuse.com/blog/a-deep-dive-into-brainwaves-brainwave-frequencies-explained-2/

12 http://www.abrahamlincolnonline.org/lincoln/speeches/fair.htm

13 https://mindmatters.ai/2020/12/spooky-action-at-a-distance-makes-sense-in-the-quantum-world/

Chapter 4

14 https://involvedmag.com/gobekli-tepe-and-the-origins-of-civilisation/

15 https://timesofindia.indiatimes.com/blogs/thedanispost/researchers-find-proof-of-ancient-atomic-war-a-great-many-years-prior/

16 https://www.universityworldnews.com/post.php?story=2015092514572690

Chapter 5

17 http://socialstudiesforkids.com/articles/ushistory/wilmarudolph.htm

Chapter 6

18 http://science.unctv.org/content/reportersblog/choices.

Chapter 7

19 https://www.psychologytoday.com/us/blog/building-the-habit-hero/202011/the-hearts-electromagnetic-field-is-your-superpower

Chapter 8

20 https://www.health.harvard.edu/newsletter_article/The_nocebo_response

21 Spiegel, H., "Nocebo: the power of suggestibility." *Preventive Medicine*, 1997. 26 (5 Pt 1): p. 616–21

Chapter 10

22 Frankl, Viktor E. *Man's Search for Meaning*. London: Rider Books, 2020.

Chapter 11

23 https: //io9. gizmodo.com/mayflies-might-just-have-the-saddest-most-perfectly-ev-5815582

24 https: //deepstash.com/idea/29096/history-of-ikigai

Made in the USA
Monee, IL
26 February 2022